The Growth of a Student-Run Pro Bono Clinic:

The Widener Physical Therapy Experience

By: Geo Derice

With Faculty and Student Board Members

Please visit www.http://chestercommunitypt.com/

for more information regarding our programs.

Instagram: theprobononetwork_

Acknowledgements:

Special thanks to Logan Sturgill and Lynne Sturgill ('07) for their editing skills.

CONTENTS

INTRODUCTION

Did you know that each year fifty percent of Americans over the age of eighteen develop a musculoskeletal injury that lasts longer than three months? That's 108 million people! Additionally, fifty-million are affected by chronic neurologic disorders such as multiple sclerosis, Parkinson disease or stroke each year. Many of these people have insurance or other resources that enable them to benefit from physical therapy. However, there is a large percentage of this injured population that does not have easy, cost-effective access to physical therapy services. (https://www.sciencedaily.com/releases/2016/03/160301114116.htm, https://onlinelibrary.wiley.com/doi/full/10.1002/ana.24897)

Can you imagine suffering an injury and you can only afford half of the treatments needed for a full recovery? Or even worse, you have no insurance, leaving you stuck with pain and limited function, but no solution in sight.

Unfortunately, this is the reality for many in Chester, Pennsylvania, a small city south of Philadelphia with a poverty rate of nearly thirty-seven percent.(datausa.io/profile/geo/chester-pa)

In this book, you will learn about one physical therapy program's initiative to make a difference. This program, when faced with the challenge of meeting the rehabilitation needs of a community, wondered, "How can we afford to have a clinic?" and then quickly realized that the real question was "How can we afford NOT to have a clinic?" The answer to this last question begins the journey of Widener University's pro bono physical therapy clinic.

This book will give insights on this start-up, their journey, and what the university anticipates for the future.

If you are a school with a physical therapy program, or a school that currently has a pro bono physical therapy clinic, THIS BOOK is certainly for you. If you are someone who wants to know how to engage physical therapy students on a higher level to promote leadership and proficiency in the application of physical therapy, THIS BOOK is for you. Are you looking for new ideas to improve your physical therapy pro bono service? THIS BOOK is also for you. And, finally, if you are newly appointed to serve on the Student Board of the Chester Community Physical Therapy Clinic at Widener University, THIS BOOK is for you!

May you learn more about the evolution of this endeavor as you prepare to guide this project into the future...

How This Book Came to Be?

This book would not have happened without Jon Herting PT, DPT ('12). You see, Jon graduated from Widener University's physical therapy program where he served on the Student Board—the group of student leaders that run the physical therapy pro bono clinic. When enlisting the services of my company (20/20 Living Inc.) to help publish his first book, *The Bodyweight Training Encyclopedia*, Jon thought it would be a great idea to connect me with Jill Black, PT, DPT, EdD. Dr. Black was the faculty advisor to the Chester Community Physical Therapy Clinic and a mentor to Jon.

Since the inception of the pro bono clinic in 2009, a growing list of schools have contacted Widener for guidance on how best to run a pro bono physical therapy clinic. The thought was, why not put together a book that covers the challenges and successes of the Widener clinic experience?

On November 20th, 2016 I talked to Jill and she agreed this book would be a great idea. She wanted the incoming physical therapy students to understand the history and growth of this project. She wanted the students to appreciate the effort and energy that previous student leaders breathed into this project, as well as understand how they too could contribute.

In essence, this book was a response to a need. The practice of simply responding to a need would become a guiding principle of how decisions were and are made at the clinic.

Real-life examples, and not just theories, of what does and does not work in a pro bono setting are included in this book. The content is designed to ensure that you are able to develop strategies which can be implemented within your own physical therapy programs.

You will learn:

+ That passionate students are the lifeblood of a successful pro bono clinic.

+ How both the faculty and student leaderships' unique approach help increase student engagement and student responsibility in the program.

+ What prompts physical therapy students who have graduated from Widener University to stay engaged with the Clinic.

...and so much more.

This is a book full of information and inspiration that will change your physical therapy program.

Now I know you might be thinking, *"I know quite a bit about running a clinic or a pro bono clinic,"* and you might also be thinking, *"Why is this guy Geo writing the book and not someone who was actually there in the trenches?"*

Let's address each of those questions.

Will you Learn Something New?

Let's address this question right now using an incredible book called *Mindset* by Carol Dweck.

In her book, Dweck explains the difference between a growth mindset and a fixed mindset. A fixed mindset believes learning is limited, while a growth mindset believes what can be learned is endless. We might compare this philosophy to being a "sponge" versus being a "rock."

If you are someone who believes you have nothing else to learn, this book is not for you. In this sense, your learning is fixed, and you are essentially a "rock." This does not make you a bad person; it just means that the possibility of learning something new is not easily achieved. If you ask me, this is a bit of a boring mindset to have.

However, if you are a "sponge," and you're interested in soaking up new things and adopting what Dweck calls a growth mindset, you are in for quite the treat. Without a doubt there will be something new in this book for you; even information in this book with which you are already familiar might hit you from a different angle, or it may prompt you to recall something you had forgotten or overlooked in the past.

Why Should I Listen to You?

If this question popped into your mind, I do not blame you. While my only personal experience with physical therapy was a few sessions for my lower back after suffering an injury weight lifting for football, I came to this topic without any preconceived notions. I was not a physical therapy student, nor did I know much about the Widener program prior to my initial discussions with Jon.

I, for one, thought I would have no interest in learning about pro bono physical therapy clinics until I met the wonderful people behind the creation of the clinic at Widener University. It's only after engaging in conversations with program directors, faculty, students, and graduates that I realize how amazing this story really is and how privileged I am to have this opportunity to convey it to others.

I want to share a secret with you which I believe demonstrates my fascination with what I learned putting this book together: I interviewed over thirty people for this book; each interview was originally scheduled for five to ten minutes in length. I was only able to do one of those thirty plus interviews in that time frame. I enjoyed it so much that I went over the scheduled time consistently! The only one that was just five minutes merely happened because we got cut off due to bad reception. And then we did another call, which lasted almost an hour!

What you're reading is an unbiased perspective of the journey to building a pro bono physical therapy clinic and why you should consider creating one at your institution. If you are already providing pro bono services, you will gain tips to enhance what you're already doing from the inspiration of the founding fathers and mothers of this incredible program at Widener University.

Dr. Jill Black, a large reason this program is where it is today, contributed incredible insights to this book. She provided many details which enabled me to share this story from my perspective.

This is my promise to you: you are about to embark on an enjoyable read. While many people might view non-fiction as something boring, this book will be anything but that. You will chuckle; your jaw will drop at times, as mine did when I heard these stories first hand; and you will be fueled to leave your imprint on physical therapy and society. I promise it will be a worthwhile read that is both informative and inspirational.

Check your bags, fasten your seatbelts, and enjoy the ride!

CHAPTER 1:
THE BIG IDEA

Apple. Google. Microsoft. Uber. Lyft. Snapchat.

Instagram. Facebook.

These are all companies that each of us has interacted with at some point in our lives, and chances are you just finished using a device, posted something on social media, or arrived home in what formerly was known as a cab.

What interests me more than anything else is how these great companies come to be. All are superstar companies in their own rights, but what were these companies like before they became what they are today?

A lot can be learned from seeing a company at the birthing stages. What inspired the idea? Were there any obstacles to starting the idea? Who were the founders of the idea? Why did the idea come out at that specific time and not at another period of time? There are so many questions, but the answers to those questions can become blueprints for other companies to follow on the road to their own success.

When I came across what was happening at Widener University's student-run physical therapy pro bono clinic, I felt compelled to speak to some of the founding partners to learn their story. I had heard of the term *pro bono* before. The law profession espouses offering services *pro bono publico*, or "for the public good."(https://www.americanbar.org/groups/legal_education/resources/pro_bono.html) But I had not heard of pro bono clinics that were run by students, nor in physical therapy.

The student-run physical therapy clinic that is the focus of this book is the Chester Community Physical Therapy Clinic. The clinic provides physical therapy services to uninsured and underinsured community members who would not otherwise be able to receive services. The clinic started on September 15, 2009 and was launched by students with faculty oversight.

I had a chance to sit down with Dr. Kerstin Palombaro, an Associate Professor and Community Engagement Coordinator in the Institute for Physical Therapy Education at Widener University and one of the faculty members instrumental in launching the clinic.

In the Fall of 2008, Dr. Kerstin Palombaro along with Dr. Jill Black began to investigate the feasibility of starting a faculty-run pro bono clinic on the edge of campus. Widener physical therapy students had already been serving at a pro bono clinic in Philadelphia, embracing the University's mission of service; however, students were interested in helping the community surrounding the university. Thus, Kerstin and Jill proceeded to conduct a community needs assessment. They interviewed and surveyed local physical therapy practices and hospital systems to explore the need for a campus-based pro bono clinic, as well as assess how receptive area clinicians would be to such a concept. Kerstin and Jill wanted to communicate clearly that the proposed clinic's intent was to be a resource and not a competitor.

The assessment revealed that area clinicians were both supportive of the idea and they recognized need. Clinicians recounted how they often would have clients exhaust their insurance benefit before achieving optimal gains. They also acknowledged that sometimes they had to turn clients away due to lack of insurance coverage.

Having confirmed a necessity for a local pro bono clinic, Kerstin and Jill turned their attention to the logistics of setting up and running such a clinic. Jill had been the director of outpatient clinics in the past, and had experience with pro bono service internationally, but did not have experience specific to pro bono services in the United States. Kerstin had experience providing pro bono service in communities, but not specifically in a clinic setting. They decided that rather than trying things from scratch, they would seek to learn from what others had already done.

In their search, they discovered a conference sponsored by the Society for Student-Run Free Clinics. The conference was not specifically for physical therapy programs but focused more on medical clinics. It was scheduled for March 2009 in Omaha, Nebraska. Dr. Robin Dole, Associate Dean and Director of the Institute for Physical Therapy Education at Widener at the time, was able to support their attendance. Kerstin and Jill also asked if there would be funds for a few students to attend and Robin said she would make it happen.

At the time, the thought was NOT that the students would be running the clinic, but rather that the students would come along and share their thoughts and ideas. As you will read, that limitation didn't constrain the creativity of Amber Cunningham ('10) and Beth Sander ('10), the two second-year students who volunteered to attend.

Professional conferences are often stimulating, but in this particular case there were some things about this conference that were less then appealing—such as being held in Nebraska in March where it was freezing cold. Jill and Kerstin knew that the two students were not coming along for a sunny vacation, but rather were strongly committed to the idea. Despite how cold it was on the outside, the conference on the inside was warm and engaging. Medical students sharing their experiences of leading free clinics left quite the impression on Kerstin and Jill, as well as Amber and Beth.

Jill now admits that she watched the medical students present with great poise and confidence and doubted that her students were capable of the same. She wondered what was inherently different in the medical students compared to her physical therapy students. She readily admits today how wrong she was in those assumptions and now realizes her students just needed the appropriate platform, and that she needed to get out of their way!

Amber and Beth also saw the poised and confident medical students but had no doubt in their capabilities to do the same. During the conference they were collectively planning and strategizing how they would return to Widener and offer a student-run model for the proposed pro bono clinic. They considered the leadership positions that would be required and were already deciding which position would be the best fit for their service and identifying fellow classmates who would be good for additional roles.

On a break in between sessions, they shared with their faculty members, a leadership organizational chart that was taking shape in their minds. Jill and Kerstin exchanged glances. The two students had apparently not gotten the message that they were along solely to provide input to the planning of the *faculty-run* pro bono clinic, not necessarily to create a *student-run* clinic. Jill expressed some caution aloud but was interrupted by the need to move to the next session. Amber and Beth were not deterred by Jill's spoken warning, and continued to grow in enthusiasm for a student-run physical therapy model throughout the remainder of the conference

On the flight home, during a layover in Ohio, Amber and Beth presented the refined leadership organizational model they had crafted to Kerstin and Jill. They also identified which roles they wished to play and who from their class might be good to fill the others. They provided strong rationale and commitment even when Jill and Kerstin told them they would not get any credit for these activities—the clinic would need to be in addition to their responsibilities as Doctor of Physical Therapy (DPT) students. This condition did not squelch their enthusiasm.

In that Ohio airport food court, Kerstin and Jill looked at one another after the students presented their idea and they were impressed. However, they were also concerned that the faculty had charged them to pursue the possibilities of a faculty-run clinic, NOT a student-run clinic! What would the faculty say when they presented this in their faculty meeting the next day? Did they really think the students could handle this? Wasn't it just last week the faculty were discussing a number of professional issues they were seeing in the students? Could these same students step-up and take on this huge professional endeavor?

Kerstin and Jill were not sure the answers to these questions, but they quietly consulted with one another and decided to align themselves with the students. Up until the call to board the plane home, they refined the model that Beth and Amber had created and made some suggestions to help strengthen it for presentation to faculty.

The groups swell of enthusiasm and excitement was countered by feelings of caution. After all, a student-run clinic was not something that the faculty were considering. When I asked Jill what she studied that helped her to come up with the idea of letting students run the show, she replied, "Geo, this wasn't my idea and I didn't study anything." This blew me away. I thought for sure she had read a series of John Maxwell books on leadership, or maybe stumbled upon an inspiring TED talk.

This simply was not the case.

The concepts of a student-run clinic, and even attending the Nebraska conference, would not have occurred if it were not for something that happened earlier. The Widener physical therapy program was preparing for this journey even before the conference, but perhaps they didn't know it. In the prior few years, the program had increased student involvement in the local community and was getting their feet wet with helping people and empowering students.

This community engagement started back with the Freedom Baptist Church after-school children's program. What started as an assigned project for a DPT course turned into a sustainable program because the students recognized a community need.

Previously, service projects were solely focused on the university body. One student attended a community volunteer fair at Widener and gathered information about several community groups that might make great partners for the Institute for Physical Therapy Education. This led to partnerships with Freedom Baptist Church, Stinson Tower, and other groups where students met an identified need to fulfill their requirements for a semester-long project for a DPT class. Students and faculty were beginning to realize that there was a whole community outside of Widener's campus where they could learn and serve.

At the end of the semester, however, students wanted to continue working with the children at Freedom Baptist Church and the other sites. They recognized that the needs of the community continued beyond the semester, and they saw the value in continuing the experience.

So, Kerstin creatively posed an elective course for the interested physical therapy students. Now, the students were able to continue their service and get academic credits. At that time, the students didn't pay tuition by the course, so this did not add to their tuition. Attaching the experience to a course allowed the participating students' continued liability coverage under the university's policy and the student's service-learning bug continued to grow.

In addition to the work at Freedom Baptist Church, they continued to offer physical activity programming at Stinson Tower, a low-income residence for senior citizens who are visually impaired and have mobility challenges.

As you can see, prior to the clinic ever being born, the wheels that would drive this big idea were already in motion, and eventually, community partners and leaders from both Freedom Baptist Church and Stinson Tower would become valuable members of the Clinic Advisory Board. This early collaboration with community members would pave the foundation for later partnerships.

Simultaneously, Jill was allowing students to serve at the Mercy Pro Bono Clinic in West Philadelphia in lieu of an assignment for one of her classes. The Mercy Pro Bono Clinic had been well-established, running out of an already existing hospital outpatient facility in the evenings. Several area physical therapy programs had their students serving there. The Widener DPT students who elected to go there came back enthusiastic about the learning experience, so more and more of their classmates started to sign up as well.

While working in the Mercy Clinic, students started noting how the demographics in West Philadelphia mirrored the demographics and needs of Chester—the community in which Widener University is located. They began to question why they were going all the way to West Philadelphia, where other Philadelphia area programs were already serving, when there were just as many needs for services in their own backyard. The students were emphatic and boldly asked: "Why aren't we doing this for Chester?"

Within this backstory, there are a few key lessons: Often, we believe that the stroke of genius comes in a very specific package, but that was not the case here. Ideas come from many different places, but inspiration requires us to be aware of what is happening and be driven by curiosity.

These students had a lot of questions and felt comfortable enough to go ahead and ask them out loud. It is one thing to see what should happen or what could happen, but if those thoughts only remain in one's mind, no one can act upon them or propose additional questions to make the idea become a reality.

It most certainly was not easy to go ahead and build a student-run physical therapy pro bono clinic. A case report published in 2011, Volume 91, Issue 11 in the journal *Physical Therapy* details the many challenges that came with the process. In my conversations with the faculty, I could sense how challenging it was to let go of the reins and allow students to lead. At the same time, I also sensed their joy and excitement in providing students an opportunity to meet the needs of their community while growing in leadership, clinical skills, and professionalism.

The environment is also important when it comes to innovation. Out of the box ideas do not happen inside a box. As you read earlier, it was attendance at the conference that helped show that this model of a student-run pro bono clinic was possible. Conferences and professional meetings can serve as a great opportunity to learn from others, ask questions to engage more in learning, and produce even better ideas. The fact that two faculty members along with two students went to the student run conference for Student-Run Free Clinics was instrumental. I do not know if the students would have built the enthusiasm to draw up a game plan during a layover if they were not exposed to what other students demonstrated was possible.

If the opportunity to go to conferences is available, I would encourage you to do so. The Widener students who run the clinic, also now organize a conference. You'll read more about that later and, of course, learn the back-story of how that came about.

As we transition from where the idea started to the actual launch of the idea, it's worth noting that great things do not have to come from a lightning bolt moment. They can come just by being aware and open to what is happening around you—and realizing that before anything can become big, it must start small. Even the largest snowstorms start off as a small snowflake. It's the consistency of small things done well, time and time again, that will often create the opportunities for larger things.

Here is something to know: While today we stand and see what the Widener experience has become, even those who were there in the beginning had no clue it would be what it is today.

Do not let the fear of failing stop you from ever taking flight. We are on the runaway now, the bags are on the plane, and we have a tank full of gas for the journey we are about to take. Let nothing, even uncertainty, stop you from moving forward. The clarity you are seeking only comes from doing, not just from thinking about it or having an idea. We must be willing to go beyond the idea and turn it into action. This is where the magic happens.

CHAPTER 2:
LETTING GO

Can anyone think of the phrase "Let It Go" without thinking of the movie *Frozen*? Letting go of anything is not easy. For many reasons, we hang onto things. Some of those reasons may be justified, but in other instances, hanging on does more harm than good. Why do you believe people hold onto things? When was the last time you were reluctant to let go of something?

If you want an example of what letting go is like, consider a parent dropping off their child at daycare for the first time. This is a vivid depiction of what letting go is like. Tears may fall and the parent might experience anxiety and an overwhelming sense of uneasiness. This scenario is revisited again when a parent lets go and allows their young adult to drive a car on their own, and then repeats again when they are letting them go to college. Does anyone remember what that was like?

I can remember being set free to drive to college on my own. It was such a freeing feeling for me. I cannot say the same for my parents. I'm sure they were worried. But as I drove there and returned home without incident, I expect the feeling of "he can do it" took over.

I imagine the Widener faculty experienced similar emotions when they went from a faculty-run clinic model to a student-run clinic model. I can recall my conversation with Jill about letting go:

> Geo: Jill, I have to know what was it really like letting go?
>
> Jill: "It was super hard to let go at first. And we didn't let go completely all at once. We took baby steps with trusting the students in leadership. It was only as they proved themselves that we relaxed

and let out the reigns a bit more. At times, I found myself picking up the reigns when I saw the balls being dropped. I learned that when I stepped in to pick up something, the students naturally stepped out and I was left having to do it. I learned that I needed to empower them to handle the challenge rather than step in and handle it for them. Sometimes the students would call me out when they felt me trying to take over. I can picture a number of them in my office saying, 'Jill, this is student-run. We can handle this. Just guide us but let us do it.' This was a big lesson for me. To this day, I still have to remind myself to 'guide … don't take over.'

Geo: Did you study any particular leadership literature or have some favorite leadership model?

Jill: "I never really studied leadership literature to know exactly how one should lead a group of people, nor did I adopt a specific model of leadership. I've always enjoyed working with a group of people to make life better in some way. Sharing in projects with others who share my passions and knowing that something good is going to come for all of us is wonderful. The goal of these projects is that it is a joint effort by all constituents and stakeholders and has benefits to all. I like to get to know who the players are and encourage them to play to their strengths. I believe these efforts should be something they WANT to do rather than something compulsory."

As Jill communicated this with me, I was reminded of the mission statement for the Institute for Physical Therapy Education Center for Community Engagement that Kerstin had shared. It was a mission statement that was put together but then revised after the students brought up the fact that it did not fully summarize the mission of their community engagement activities.

Here's how the mission statement reads now:

> *The Institute for Physical Therapy Education Center for Community Engagement believes that health and wellness is a basic human right. We strive to promote health and wellness through the provision of education, resources, and services, reciprocally and collaboratively, with all stakeholders. We desire to empower and improve the communities with whom we interact.*
>
> *The mission for The Chester Community Physical Therapy Clinic specifically is to simultaneously improve healthcare access to physical therapy services by providing pro bono physical therapy services to underserved and underinsured community members while educating a new generation of physical therapists in the areas of competency, character, citizenship, and social responsibility.*

As you can see, the style of leadership, mission, and vision the Institute for Physical Therapy Education's Center for Community Engagement and The Chester Community Physical Therapy Clinic strive for is a win-win situation for all parties involved. This is an important lesson that should not be overlooked. There's no mission that is more exciting and more fulfilling than one that incorporates all parties and stakeholders. As you think about building out your mission statement and the style of leadership required to build a successful organization, remember that all stakeholders should benefit.

Back to my conversation with Jill. She also shared her belief that when you have a clear vision of what needs to be done, it's all about having folks that want the same in your corner. Never build a foundation on people that don't want to be there or are forced to be there. This kind of culture creates a poor work environment and stunts future growth. Those who don't engage the vision become bad weeds that choke up the entire garden. When you have people CHOOSING to participate in the mission, amazing things can happen.

The next step is helping people identify their strengths and helping them find the place where their strengths can truly shine. Letting go can often be perceived as doing less, but this is not the case when done well. Faculty have an important role in learning where students thrive, identifying when they need assistance, and deciding when to allow them to stretch, as well as knowing when to step in.

The student-run model does come with its challenges, and one of the ways to help ease those challenges is by having an open-door policy. When speaking with Jill, she shared with me how important it is to her that the students feel comfortable coming into her office to share how things are going and pitch their ideas. She acknowledged that there are times when she encourages them to reshape their ideas because it's been done in the past and therefore there were key lessons learned that could benefit the students in the present. Experience is invaluable. With access to history, you are able to provide context for the students so they can make better and more effective choices. It's not so much a major shift, but just a tweak that is often needed to take ideas from "no way!" to "let's give that a try." The open-door policy helps break down barriers between students and faculty and helps foster germination of some of the best ideas.

A great deal of the success in this model requires getting out of the way of the students. Stepping back creates a vacuum that the students have an opportunity to fill. Many do not realize this, but for someone to rise to the occasion, someone else (such as a faculty member) might need to get out of the way. Remember how Jill first thought that the medical students were poised and polished and professional and her students were not? Once she realized that the faculty needed to get out of the way and allow the students opportunities, she understood that they were just as poised, polished, and professional. They could certainly do it. They just needed to be given the chance.

Another similar and vital element is open communication. We've all heard that communication is the key to any relationship, and that is also true with the relationship between faculty and students in the student-run model. Often times, when stepping in, students might feel as if you are telling them they are wrong or to step back. Without communication they will not step back in. Many times, all we want to do as faculty is provide that spark or that one-degree redirect that is needed, but it is important to communicate that with the students. This helps them feel like the project and work is theirs, giving them ownership. When they are owners of the work, they find it more important and pour themselves into it.

Giving ownership also shows students that you trust them. This is another key element to any successful relationship. Without trust, no one feels empowered and the fear of having to be perfect produces more mistakes. An effective model enables students to make choices and best prepares them to become strong professionals and leaders in their field. The faculty's role is simply to provide guidance so that the student choices are the best they can be.

Perhaps I've overlooked a question you might now be asking as you read this. You might think, "How persuasive were the students who helped lead this idea for a clinic?" The answer depends on whom you are asking. From the students' perspective, not much convincing was necessary. Amber, one of the initial conference-goers, felt that Jill and Kerstin did not need much convincing to adopt the student-led model. She believed that Jill and Kerstin thought the model was best suited for the needs of the university, the physical therapy program, and the community at the time.

From the perspective of the faculty, Kerstin and Jill noted that it was with trepidation that they brought the student proposal to the faculty meeting. They weren't confident this was a good idea, and they weren't sure of their faculty's response. After much discussion in the Monday afternoon faculty meeting following the Omaha conference, the faculty voted to allow the students to give it a try but charged Jill and Kerstin to keep a close watch on them. No one was sure it would succeed.

What lessons can we pull from how the student-run model came about?

If you are faculty reading this, "letting go" was the overarching theme of this chapter, but other points emerged as well.

For starters, the previous work of the students in the community and at the West Philadelphia pro bono clinic prepared the students and the faculty to consider this next step of empowering student leadership in the creation of a student-run pro bono clinic. Always examine what direction your program is going or has gone to see what might fit best for your next step.

Another important factor is the significance of trusting your students. As we stated earlier, very few relationships succeed without trust. Following that is the importance of communication. Clearly communicating thoughts, ideas, events, frustrations, and hopes is very important. Without communication, it's fair to assume both faculty and students would have grown frustrated and potentially unsuccessful.

CHAPTER 3:
ALL HANDS ON DECK

The beginning of this chapter is going to sound a bit cliché.

"Rome was not built in a day" is the common refrain whenever someone lacks the patience to follow the process in a complex undertaking. In fact, at the time of writing this book, the Philadelphia 76ers' team slogan is "Trust the Process." The faculty and students of this clinic might have adopted the same slogan because "Trust the Process" was something they really had to embody right from the start.

After the faculty voted to allow the students to take the lead, Beth and Amber wasted no time in presenting the leadership opportunity to their classmates. Their model involved positions with responsibilities for running certain aspects of the clinic. In March of 2009, they developed an application that interested classmates could complete and had Jill and Kerstin help them decide who should serve in which position. Once their Class of 2010 had members named to the Student Board, they reached out to the class below them and distributed applications. The Class of 2010 Student Board helped select the Class of 2011 Student Board. Both Student Boards gathered and discussed a timeline for the clinic opening. They visited a potential space that had been identified for the clinic and discussed obstacles and needs with Kerstin and Jill. The Student Board decided they would like to open the doors on September 15, 2009, and that was just six months away.

The space available was approximately seven-hundred square feet which had been a motion analysis and gait lab located within an old stone home about five blocks from the campus physical therapy building. The two-story house had once belonged to a local family physician who had his office there. Upon his death, he bequeathed the home to Widener University. In addition to the old motion analysis lab, the house was also the home of Widener's Neuropsychological Assessment Center.

The motion analysis lab had not been used for some time. When the students first entered, they encountered cobwebs and a musty odor. The floor and walls were black, and the space was filled with junk. Six months did not seem like sufficient time to get this place ready.

Faculty contacted University Operations and requested that the walls be painted white. The Operations Department also put up walls to allow for a small office space within the square room. Students worked to clear out the junk and began to build a relationship with their neighbors in the Neuropsychology Assessment Center. A quick assessment for ADA compliance demonstrated a great LACK of compliance. Faculty realized they could put in for a University Capital Improvement Grant to widen the front door and make the entrance to the house accessible. This grant would also provide accessible parking spaces. They were successful in obtaining the grant and the work was completed that summer.

There was a black spongy floor in the gait lab and that was undesirable for the clinic floor. In May, the Class of 2009 left a graduation gift check with enough money to buy new laminate flooring materials, but not enough money to pay for the installation. The father of one of the students from the Class of 2010 was a carpenter and offered to come in on the weekend and do it for free! A prior gift from the Class of 2008, which had been designated to help the idea of developing a clinic, was finally used to purchase the clinic's first two plinths.

In researching the best deal on plinths, Jill spoke to Mr. Michael Couliandis, owner of M.A. Rallis Rehabilitation Equipment. Michael was moved by the story of the students creating a clinic to serve community members who would otherwise not receive services and offered to sell them the plinths at cost. Not only that, he offered to sell them anything they needed at cost. The students began a "wish list" of items and as donated funds came in, they called Michael to see what items they could purchase next. In this way, they were able to outfit the space with new equipment rather than older equipment that might have needed repair. Faculty also pulled together funds to purchase cubicle curtains and track. An alumnus fundraising event yielded funds to purchase things like ankle weights, dumb bells, and a movable mirror rack. Students had artwork brought in for the clinic walls. Amanda Reinmiller ('11) painted a mural on one wall. Jess Darrah ('10) sewed client gowns and curtain valances for the windows.

There were students who even created their own equipment. Wayne Burkholtz ('10), was a student with many skills and might as well be called Mr. Home Improvement. In addition to building a slant board and racks for weights and physio balls, he also installed ceiling eyebolts for overhead pulleys. However, his signature contribution was a plinth he made himself. Never having built one before, he copied those in the lab, purchased the lumber and upholstery, brought in the tools, and constructed it. It is the sturdiest of all plinths to date. To see what the clinic looks like now compared to the beginning is unbelievable. Building the Clinic truly was an all hands on deck approach.

Preparing the physical space was one challenge, but setting up the operational pieces such as documentation and marketing materials was yet another. Amber Cunningham, as the 2010 Outcomes Coordinator, took on the initial start-up documentation paperwork. If you are old enough, you might remember what it was like to take pictures with a camera that required film. Today digital cameras make quick work of that process and we can't imagine a world without them. At the pro-bono clinic things ran pretty "old school" at the beginning. Amber shared how they started with paper documentation and client charts. With notes from class and samples from an area clinic, she put together the templates for all of the paper documentation forms. While most clinics were making transitions to electronic medical records, the clinic had to start simply and paper was the way to do it.

Aaron Peffer, Class of 2011 Marketing Officer, took on the creation of the clinic marketing materials, which included informational flyers for various audiences (physicians, clients, and alumni donors), prescription pads, business cards, and appointment cards. Some of these items required approval from the University Relations Department and he learned to navigate their approval process. Crystal Ayers, Class of 2010 Operations Coordinator, put her organizational skills to work and created a system to identify where all things were kept. Parts of her system are still in use eight years later.

Many people wait until everything is exactly perfect to begin, but what I personally loved when listening to these humble beginnings was the fact that there was no waiting for ideal or perfect conditions to move forward. Many dreams never come true, and many bold ideas are never realized because we are led to believe that all the ducks must be in a row before beginning. This mentality leaves ideas lazily sitting on the couch waiting for an epiphany moment that never seems to come.

The trick was to have enough of the important pieces in place to start. The students wanted to make a great first impression on the community. They recognized that one bad experience could quickly taint their reputation and they sought to have as many of the essential pieces in place to get off to a good start. Many additions and improvements, though, were made after the initial opening. In fact, each new group of students that enters the Institute for Physical Therapy Education and steps into Student Board leadership roles find new ways to improve upon the clinic, to better serve clients, and to leave a legacy of their own on this ever-growing and changing project.

CHAPTER 4:
OPENING THE DOORS

When you have a great idea, the assumption is that the floodgates open and people are lining up around the corner looking to participate. This, unfortunately, isn't how most companies or organizations start; but we never hear those stories unless the founders decide to write a book about their process. I'm reminded of Howard Schultz, who tells the story of how Starbucks started. Schultz faced rejection many times as he tried to bring an overseas concept to America. Thanks to Schultz's perseverance, you can find a Starbucks on college campuses and on practically every other corner in both major and smaller cities.

This same perseverance was needed when the pro bono clinic doors opened with only one client scheduled. Incidentally, that client was not even from the community the students expected to serve. This is like buying chocolates, flowers, and a nice gift for your valentine only to have that special someone call out sick and be unable to come to dinner. For students like Amber Cunningham ('10), Beth Sander ('10) and Wayne Burkholtz ('10), there were many humbling events that required persistence, resilience, and patience to endure.

Wayne recalls that their first client was a two-month-old baby with torticollis, a condition the students had not yet learned to treat. They had not had their pediatrics course yet! The physical therapist providing licensed supervision that night also did not have much experience in pediatrics. He remembers contacting Dr. Robin Dole, their Associate Dean and Director and a pediatric specialist, who willingly provided supervision and direction. This is an example of faculty stepping in when asked and voluntarily meeting the need.

Any organization that is going to thrive through growing pains needs this kind of support. Eight out of ten businesses fail within the first year. (https://www.forbes.com/sites/ericwagner/2013/09/12/five-reasons-8-out-of-10-businesses-fail/#4b018d246978) As a business owner myself, I know that a key cause of failure is lack of support. The Student Board did not have this issue because of the great support and help of the faculty, but this support did not mean that everything was a piece of cake in the beginning.

The clinic joyfully opened its doors that first night to receive just that one client. The following week, a second client appeared. This client was an older woman who had fractured her ankle and had been receiving therapy at a local physical therapy clinic, but she soon maxed out her cap of services allowed by Medicare. Her therapist was an alumnus of the Widener University physical therapy program and had heard about the opening of the clinic. So now the students were eagerly working with two clients at the extremes of the lifespan.

In the beginning, the clinic was open just two evenings a week, and treated only two clients for the first few months. After four months with their client population growing, they chose to open a third night. After six months, a fourth night was added.

In the second year, their client base continued to grow, but the student leaders were adamant that they didn't want to have a waiting list. They assessed their resources. One of the solutions they implemented is described fully in a later chapter about space. The first space expansion that was done effectively doubled the space and doubled the number of clients that could be seen. The doubling of clients can be seen in the statistics for year three and four. See Figure 1.

The number of client visits made another big jump in the fifth year, causing a dilemma for the student leadership. One of the reasons for the increase was related to determining which clients were ready for discharge, but there was no clear or consistent path to accomplish this efficiently. This time, rather than trying to increase space (options for that were relatively non-existent anyway), they considered how they might improve care and progression to discharge. This led to the institution of *care teams* and Grand Rounds, both of which you will read more about in a later chapter. This initiative not only improved the student and client experience, but also led to more efficient progression of care and timely discharge.

The numbers became more manageable in year six. However, years seven, eight, and now nine show a strong upward trend again and the current student leadership is working on the next solution.

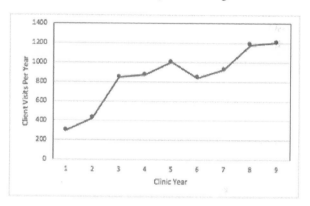

Figure 1. Growth in number of client visits over time.

Additional Challenge and Improvements

Remember that paper documentation process? The paper system filled the need at the time but was not ideal as more and more healthcare systems were turning to EMR or "Electronic Medical Record" systems. But such systems can be expensive, especially for a pro bono operation. Wayne Burkholtz ('10), while attending a conference, visited the WebPT exhibit booth and discussed the possibility of having WebPT donate use of their system. WebPT had developed one of the first physical therapy specific electronic documentation systems. While they were not willing to donate the entire system, they were willing to allow the clinic to use their educational version, which was at a significantly reduced cost. Wayne was nearing graduation as this took shape, so he passed his WebPT connections on to his first-year physical therapy student roommate, Jon Herting. Jon was the Class of 2012 Community Relations and Marketing Officer and he continued the dialogue with WebPT. Soon WebPT was up and operational in the clinic. To support active use of the WebPT system, donations had come in to enable the purchase of eight iPads and the Widener IT department worked to enhance the capabilities of the Wi-Fi in the clinic building.

Collecting data and information is important to any successful clinic. With these new resources the clinic was able to move away from paper for their medical documentation and for their client satisfaction surveys which were used from the very beginning of clinic operation. Eventually Georgia Spano and Kyle Bauer, both Class of 2016 Health and Wellness Coordinators, made significant improvements in the client satisfaction surveys—in both the questions that were asked and how they gathered and reported that data. They transferred the survey to the iPad for ease of completion and developed mechanisms to track the data for making suggested improvements. Asking for client feedback has been an important part of the clinic's recipe for success. Acting on the feedback they receive has led to positive changes, clinic growth, and improvement for all stakeholders.

Another subsequent improvement was the addition of a washer and dryer for the laundering of the many sheets, pillowcases, and towels used each evening. For the first two years, the student leaders took turns at a local laundromat. This required a significant amount of time and a lot of quarters! One day, a few students realized that there was a washer and dryer in the clinic basement, but they were not in working condition. Unfortunately, there was no funding for new ones.

Enter Jon Herting ... again. He understood that the clinic had a limited budget, so he went to an unlikely source for help.

While walking across campus, he saw a company truck that was servicing the washers and dryers in the campus dormitories. Jon noted the company name, address, and telephone number, and unapologetically composed a letter to the company asking if they had any extra machines that they could contribute to the clinic. He shared the vision of the clinic and the need. To his surprise, the service company offered to donate a refurbished set at no cost. This was a great lesson on not being afraid to ask. Jon understood this, and it served the clinic to have someone as bold as he to help secure things like a washer and dryer.

Pulling back the curtains on the opening and improvements made to the clinic allows us to see first-hand what the early days were like. The hope is to provide inspiration that you too can begin something even on a small scale, even without all the answers. As President Harry S. Truman noted, "Imperfect action is better than perfect inaction."

The purpose of this chapter is to show you the humble beginnings of the clinic so that you too will begin something at your school or at your organization, even if it's small. Lao Tzu, musing about success, once said: "A journey of a thousand miles must begin with a single step."

Take the first step, even if you cannot see what is coming next. All you need is a deep desire and you'll see how the answers you're looking for often follow the actions you are willing to take. Yes, that even includes actions that might seem mundane or out of your job description.

CHAPTER 5:
GETTING THE WORD OUT

Dan Kennedy, in his book *The Ultimate Marketing Plan*, poses the question:

"If you opened a hamburger restaurant, what is the first thing you need to be successful?" Most people respond with the following answers:

+ A nice looking restaurant.

+ An amazing recipe for burgers.

+ Great milkshakes to go with the burgers.

+ And lots more.

The correct response, according to marketing genius Kennedy, was a "starving crowd."

When I first read this I thought, "Duh, why didn't I think of that?"

When the clinic started, the student leaders knew they had to build awareness with their target clients. Their first attempt at getting the word out was to hold an official open house for the community to come and see the newly renovated space ready to serve their needs! The students gave the clinic one final cleaning, sent out the invitations across the Widener campus and to Chester community leaders, and even ran an advertisement in the local newspaper. They arrived early and opened the doors to receive the crowds. But there were no crowds. Throughout the evening, a number of colleagues and dignitaries from the University made an appearance, but absent were folks from the Chester community. The open house served to spread the word among the Widener community but did nothing to draw in the local residents.

From this experience, the Student Board learned that they couldn't expect the Chester community to come to them; they needed to go to the community.

The Class of 2011 researched and found that Chester hosted an annual event called Riverfest on the Delaware River waterfront. The daylong event included food, vendors, music, games, and an evening concert. During the day, community organizations were offered a booth to share information about their services. The Student Board secured one of those booths, and furnished it with a tablecloth, desktop displays, and flyers to advertise the clinic's services. And it turned out that this approach was much more effective than the open house and confirmed the need to go into the community as a partner.

Due to Pennsylvania regulations for physical therapy, students serving in the clinic can only treat clients who come in with a physician's referral, (regulations also require that they have a licensed physical therapist supervising them onsite). That meant that another marketing target was the local physicians. Reaching physicians was the task of the Community Relations and Marketing Officers for the clinic, which at the beginning included Wayne Burkholtz ('10) followed by Aaron Peffer ('11).

Cold calling at physicians' offices was one of the first and largest challenges for the Marketing Officers. As Wayne described it, "First you had to see who was willing to even listen to what you had to say. At times you would not even get a chance to speak to the physician. At best you might be able to speak to the person at the front desk." However, these challenges did not deter them as they found people were very excited about what the clinic was doing and what it represented. Sometimes their audience thought it was too good to be true and were looking for the catch. It's like someone coming up to you and saying here is a free car, wouldn't your first question be, "What's wrong with it?" Well, what was potentially "wrong" or different was that clients were treated by Physical Therapy doctoral students under the supervision of licensed Physical Therapists. Students do not have the same amount of experience, but they bring great commitment and compassion. The other misnomer that had to be corrected was that the session is not "free." The students ask for a five dollar fee for service—if the client is able to pay. If clients are not able to pay, they are not turned away, but they are expected to pay if they can. Sometimes clients even "pay" with baked goods or pizzas. The students structured the small fee for service to put a value on their service and to protect the dignity of the clients who wish to come and give what they can. *Pro bono publico* translates to "for the public good" and Widener believes that "free" isn't necessarily in the public good for a number of reasons.

Initially, the Student Board realized the hard way that not everyone in the Chester community thought fondly of Widener University. In the past, the institution had not always acted in ways that was supportive of the local community. Much of that has changed in recent years under new presidential leadership but old feelings of mistrust remained. The students recognized that they needed to work to build trust again and that the clinic was one vehicle to do that.

Slow and steady did win this race as a few people took leaps of faith and gave the clinic a try and found that the services were as advertised. The clinic encouraged them to share their experiences with others, as word of mouth is often the best marketing.

Essentially, building awareness is what marketing is all about. If you are looking to do any kind of initiative, be sure to have a marketing plan. It does not have to be a perfect marketing plan, but as long as you have one you can go ahead and make adjustments and eventually, as you continue to provide high quality service, the right people will get word of the great work you are doing and share this information with others.

Raising Funds

Another part of marketing includes fund raising, and the Student Board had dedicated fund raising positions. The clinic needed to be self-supporting. The University provided the space rent-free and provided utility coverage. The licensed physical therapists were providing supervision at no cost. The students were providing the administrative and operational functions at no cost. But funds were needed to purchase equipment, furniture, and office and clinic supplies.

Heather Wnorowski ('10) and Vanessa Kershaw ('11) were the first Fund Officers. Their first fundraiser was selling clinic T-shirts that they had designed. Unfortunately, the vendor "stretched" the Widener University logo, rendering the shirts unsellable by the Widener University Relations standards. Undeterred, they sought other avenues of fundraising.

To date, the most successful and repeated fundraising event has been a 5K race, typically in the spring. Putting together a 5K is not easy, but one of the faculty members, Dr. Sam Pierce, had experience with running these events and offered his guidance. Scott Cheney, Class of 2013 Clinic Coordinator, shared how the first year of the 5k did not have a huge turnout; however, in the second year participation grew exponentially. With experience, subsequent races became easier to organize. Each class had their specific strengths when it came to race planning. Some had more knowledge and experience about racing, others were more experienced in event planning. Over the years, the 5K race fundraiser has taken on several iterations. Fund Officer Alanna DiBiassi ('15) worked to incorporate a parallel event for the children at a local Chester elementary school.

After several years of sponsoring a traditional 5K race, Fund Officer Caitlin Grobaker ('16) decided to shift it to a "colorful run." This appealed to the larger Widener student body and infused new energy into the event. Fraternities and sororities sponsored "color stations" and their members were in charge of throwing color on the runners. This year, Fund Officers Liz Antonucci ('19) and Leo Harmon ('19) are transforming the race into a "glow-in-the-dark" run. They are calling it "Glow Crazy" and will be holding it at dusk to allow the runners to be illuminated as they run.

No matter what form the clinic's 5K fundraiser takes, the students have successfully built a strong sponsor base that return year after year to financially support their efforts. Earnings range from $6000-$8000 annually and support student attendance at a conference to represent the clinic.

Fund Officers Kasey Dietrich ('18) and Brittany Burkholder ('19) identified and instituted a number of ongoing fundraisers that they have passed on to the classes of 2019 and 2020. They include Football Mania, Wawa Hoagie coupons, and restaurant night fundraisers.

A brilliant idea for fundraising came from Physical Therapy Program Secretary, Jeanne Nolan. Jeanne is a beloved member of the Institute for Physical Therapy Education and is the key to all things running smoothly in the department. Coincidentally, she happened to start in her position the same year that the clinic opened, and she has been a strong facilitator of the students' and clinic's growth and successes. After watching the commitment of the students for the first year, a fundraising idea came to her mind. She oversees the annual graduation banquet and routinely puts together a program pamphlet for the event. Why not sell half and full-page "shout outs" to parents, friends, and family members of the graduates? She offered to advertise the opportunity in her graduation banquet mailing, collect the money and the "shout outs," and to work with Student Board members to create the program pamphlet. She started this with the graduating class of 2011 and has continued it ever since. The program routinely generates $500 - $600 a year.

Another fundraising source is the Institute for Physical Therapy Education's Continuing Education Institute, chaired by faculty member Dr. Dawn Gulick. The purpose of this Institute is to provide continuing education to alumni and to clinical instructors as well as to the wider professional community. The Continuing Education Institute plans and oversees a number of courses per year. Any profits made from these courses go directly to support the work of the clinic.

The student and faculty leaders are often asked by those creating or running clinics if they have grants supporting the clinic; the answer is no. In 2009 and 2010, grant monies were scarce, and while the clinic board successfully secured some very small ones for a few specific pieces of equipment, they did not even try for a larger one that would cover all operation expenses. They did not want to rely on a large grant that might eventually dry up. Their goal was to create an initiative that could be self-sustaining. They realized that they were making a commitment to the community as they opened the doors and they wanted to be able to be in the community for the long haul. To this end, they designed the initiative to run on a shoestring budget. The extra money they raise allows them to do bigger and better things, but if they didn't have that money, they would still be able to function. They feel this has been a key to their sustainability and success.

Over time, they have developed relationships with regular donors from Foundations, faculty or alumni, and other members of the Widener community. The Fund Officers work hard to maintain and pass down those relationships to the Fund Officers in the class below them. They send out an annual donor letter with updates on the clinic and anecdotes from clients and students giving account for the activities and accomplishments facilitated by their regular donations. In this way, they encourage a regular base of support.

Fundraising has its good, bad, and ugly parts. There are moments of desperation, and there are moments of frustration when others are not buying into your vision. However, remembering the *what* and the *why* allows you to stay in the game long enough to figure out the *how*. Be encouraged. No matter what stage you're in now, move forward with your own fundraising efforts.

"Anytime you see a turtle up on top of a fence post, you know he had some help." - Alex Haley

This is a quote I truly enjoy because it speaks to the reality of how most great feats are accomplished: With the help of others. Whether you look at the greatest athletes, the greatest artists, the greatest politicians, or the greatest companies, their successes could never happen in a vacuum. The help of others is necessary. This is no different when you are trying to answer the cry of a community. The cause may be present but without support, sustainability is not a certainty.

CHAPTER 6:
THE EVOLUTION OF THE STUDENT-RUN MODEL

Do you remember the last time you solved a puzzle? Puzzles have been around for ages and even with modern technology puzzles are still relevant today. A simple search on eBay came up with 178,476 puzzles being sold. Now, I know you might be wondering what this has to do with this book… I'm glad you asked. When it comes to completing a puzzle, what is the key you need to solve it? A model. Without knowing what the solution looks like, you are not able to duplicate it.

In this chapter we break down in detail what the model is, describe how it came about, and, more importantly, explain the changes over the years. This chapter is certain to inspire you to challenge the status quo, motivate you to create a student-run model, or stimulate thinking about how your current model can evolve. Remember, even if you are on the right track, the train will hit you if you don't move. That being said, let us dive in to the student-run model at Widener University's past and present.

I believe the student-run approach is something that had to be seen previously in some capacity before it can be duplicated. The idea of a student-run model for the clinic did not come out of nowhere. It was inspired by similar models seen when the students and faculty were able to attend the Nebraska conference. my Well, they came home with a preliminary model for the organization of the clinic that they had adapted from examples they saw at the conference. Many of the models related to medical students serving in medical free clinics, but they took what they found relevant and adjusted to fit their vision of a physical therapy student-run model. Their initial model had three major components: a faculty board, a team of licensed physical therapist supervisors, and an eight-member student board. In short order, the students expanded the board to ten members to allow for extra help in needed areas. The ten-member board is pictured in Figure 2.

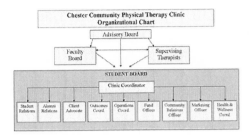

Figure 2. Early Organizational Model

The Student Board was placed in the center to emphasize their leadership. The Faculty Board and Supervising Physical Therapists were placed above, but on either side to denote their ultimate responsibility over the Student Board, and also their deference to the Student Board's ownership and leadership.

The Faculty Board initially consisted of three faculty members: Kerstin and Jill and the physical therapy program director, Dr. Robin Dole. Over time, three additional members, Mark Paterson, Ellen Erdman, and Sandy Campbell, were added to the board. Mark, an experienced clinical teacher, was brought on to facilitate mentorship of the clinical supervisors. Ellen, as an IPTE Director of Clinical Education, was added to facilitate fostering student preparations for their first full-time clinical experiences. Sandy, with a PhD in health policy, was charged with helping the Student Board to shape and expand relevant policies for the clinic.

The intent of the originators of the Faculty Board was to make more than one faculty member responsible for the success and oversight of the clinic. The originators did not want to set up this project based on the vision and energy of just one faculty member. What would happen if that faculty member moved on? They wanted broad-based institutional support to enable the clinic to endure.

The Faculty Board is responsible for the administrative oversight of the Student Board. The licensed Physical Therapist Supervisors also provide oversight of clinical care, but students perform all administrative duties in the clinic. A Student Board Clinic Administrator is assigned as the Clinic Manager for each night of care. The Clinic Administrator ensures that all administrative processes run smoothly, freeing the licensed Physical Therapists to focus solely on providing clinical oversight for physical therapy care. In the beginning, the licensed supervisors were volunteers, and consisted of faculty members or recent alumni.

A key component of the model has been that faculty are not required to participate in the clinic. They are always invited to serve, but never mandated. Amazingly, many faculty choose to serve when needed.

About three years into clinic operation, the patient visit census was growing across the four evenings of care, and the Faculty Board determined that it was time to pay a supervisor for each night of the week. Prior to this, all of the supervisors were volunteers. The program hired four supervisors and brought them on as adjunct professors. This move contributed to stability and continuity of service for all stakeholders: the students, the supervisors, and the clients. The students call the paid supervisors their "Primary Supervisors." A pool of voluntary "Secondary Supervisors" serve alongside the Primary Supervisors. Secondary supervisors typically serve once or twice a month. Currently, the students have a pool of twenty-five secondary supervisors, many of whom are alumni eager to come back and serve in the clinic.

The original Student Board consisted of eight members with the Clinic Coordinator serving as the chair. The chief role of the Clinic Coordinator has been to oversee and coordinate all activities of the Student Board as well as serve as the prime communicator with the Faculty Board and outside constituents. Here is the role of each of the other seven positions:

Position	Primary Responsibility
Student Scheduler	Scheduling classmates to serve in the clinic
Client Scheduler	Scheduling clients in the clinic
Alumni/Supervisor Scheduler	Scheduling licensed supervisors in the clinic
Operations Coordinator	Maintenance of the clinic equipment, supplies, and space
Outcomes Coordinator	Tracking of all outcomes
Fund Officer	Raising money for the clinic
Community Relations Officer	Marketing services to the community and referral sources

About three years into the clinic operation, the faculty and student leadership added a community advisory board to the model. The community advisory board consists of key members of the university, community partners' previous clients, alumni, area physical therapists, and the Student and Faculty Boards. The Advisory Board meets once each semester. The Student Board members give a presentation to the Advisory Board members, who in turn provide insight, direction, encouragement, and instruction.

Over time, the Student Board model has evolved. After just a few years, it became apparent that the Community Relations Officer was a very big job. Hence, the position divided into two: the Referral Marketing Officer and the Social Media/Community Relations Officer. In addition, a Health and Wellness Coordinator position was added. This position was charged with helping clients discharge and integrate back into the community. Titles of positions have changed over time to better capture their roles and each year the Student Board members review and revise the bylaws to capture the evolution of their roles.

As the clinic grew, and the student leadership began to share their experiences with others, they created both a Pro Bono Network and a Pro Bono National Honor Society. Both of these entities were the vision of two members of the Class of 2014. As these new groups grew, the Student Board created the student leadership positions of National Conference Chair and Pro Bono National Honor Society Officer. The Class of 2015 championed both of these positions and developed a website to promote them. The Class of 2015 also created the role of Clinic Administrator and was the first class to don blue dress shirts when representing the clinic and the Pro Bono Network at National Conferences.

Another change was made three years ago in an attempt to better clarify what is meant by a "student-run" clinic. Students and faculty realized that some had the misconception that "student-run" meant that students were handling all aspects of the clinic, including client care. This is not and has never been the case. The students are running the administrative aspects of the clinic, aspects that do not require a physical therapy license. Students are providing physical therapy care in the clinic but are doing so under the supervision of licensed Physical Therapists in compliance with the State Practice Act. In addition, more than just the Student Board leadership were providing care in the clinic. With the Class of 2015, all Doctor of Physical Therapy (DPT) students started spending time in the clinic. An organizational box was added to the model to delineate that all of the student Physical Therapists are providing care under the oversight of licensed Physical Therapists. See Figure 3.

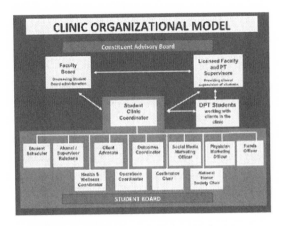

Figure 3. Organizational Model

CHAPTER 7:
BEYOND CHESTER

What do you think of when you read the following?

Las Vegas.

Gambling, glitz, shows, and no state income tax? How about "What happens In Vegas, stays in Vegas"? A saying that encourages keeping secrets...

Keeping secrets was not what took place in Chester as news about the clinic and students began to spread, first locally and, as you will read, nationally.

As the clinic began receiving more inquiries from other universities, the students realized that others might benefit from the formation of a network—a forum for student leaders to connect with other programs, address common questions, share tips, and learn from one another's challenges and solutions. Students started the network as just an e-mail chain to provide a place for open communication. Schools were encouraged to ask questions and share ideas. It was a virtual network no different than what you might find in a group on Facebook.

Brian Kennedy, Class of 2015 Clinic Coordinator, identified the need to have a web presence and pursued setting up a website up for the clinic. He also designed a postcard which advertised free webinars to schools who wanted to consult with the Student Board team. Since then, a number of Student Boards have made virtual connection with many schools to answer their questions and offer suggestions. Sometimes, students from other programs travel to take a tour of the clinic and meet with Student Board members in person. Temple University is one of those programs that made the local visit. Two enthusiastic students and a supportive faculty member came to tour the clinic and meet with student and faculty leaders. A year later, Temple launched its own student-run pro bono clinic serving the uninsured and underinsured of North Philadelphia. Widener's Student Board was thrilled to be invited to the ribbon cutting ceremony!

Contacts from other universities were only one example of the clinic's impact outside of Chester, but it is important to remember that making an impact beyond Chester was not the intention of the clinic at first. Their initial focus was doing the best job they could in the Chester community. What happened next illustrates a principle of the late Walt Disney: "Whatever you do, do it well. Do it so well that when people see you do it, they will want to come back and see you do it again and they will want to bring others and show them how well you do what you do." This is what was happening at the clinic at Widener. The students were doing what they did so well that others heard about it and wanted to learn more. When looking to build influence and impact, it is important to start with doing what you do well; the rest, as they say, is history.

From the very beginning, Jill and Kerstin were committed to sending students to conferences to learn more and to report on their own work. You may remember that it was in 2009 that students first attended the Student-Run Conference for Student-Run Clinics in Omaha. By the time that conference rolled around in February of 2010, the clinic had started, and now Beth Sander ('10), Amber Cunningham ('10), Wayne Burkholtz ('10), and others returned to that conference with a poster to display and share their work; but also with a thirst to learn more. In time, the Student Board sent representation to more conferences, some of them local, some regional, and some national. For the most part, every Student Board member has had an opportunity to travel and represent the clinic at a conference. It was after attending some of these conferences that Christina Guay, Class of 2014 Clinic Coordinator, championed an idea.

Christina attended many conferences as part of her extracurricular activities while she was in graduate school. By attending conferences, she learned how they ran, and even participated in the conferences by giving presentations and serving on a conference board. When I spoke with her, she shared with me how invaluable the experiences were in developing her management skills, something physical therapy students, especially those who run clinics, would need. She felt the experience helped her become more professional and shaped her career path.

In late 2012, Christina returned from presenting at the American Physical Therapy Association (APTA) National Student Conclave. She was moved by the many questions that she received after the presentation and realized there was a real desire for more information. When she returned from Winter break in January of 2013, she came to Jill and asked, "Why don't we hold our own conference here?" Jill responded that she thought the idea had potential and that perhaps it was something to consider for 2014. Christina was adamant. She was convinced it could happen in March of 2013—just two months away. Putting together a conference, however, was not easy. As with starting the clinic, the students and faculty did not have all the answers. What they did know was there was a need for a space where physical therapy students working in pro bono clinics could share their challenges, concerns, and innovative ideas to help one another.

With a short time to plan, Jeanne Nolan, the Program Secretary, made a call to Widener room reservations and learned that a conference room was available for just one Saturday in March. Christina asked her to book it and proceeded to have the Student Board make advertising materials to distribute when a cohort of board members attended a national physical therapy professional conference in San Diego the next month.

Realistically, Christina and her board hoped that at least twenty to twenty-five people might attend from some of the Philadelphia area schools. When speaking with the students, they acknowledged that they did not expect to draw a large attendance this first time. Much to their surprise, the conference drew seventy-eight attendees representing sixteen different programs. They realized then that their intuition was right: There was a need to network around student-run pro bono clinics and an annual conference would help meet that need. Upon the heels of the 2013 conference, they set a date for March of 2014 and started planning.

They strategized tweaks in the conference program such as breakout sessions to help maximize the experience and allow for attendee participation. The first conference had just one track of sessions, but they planned for two for the next conference. Instead of listening to long talks on topics that may or may not be of interest, the additional breakout sessions would give attendees choices and opportunities to present themselves. From the start, the conference planners were committed to allowing time for networking and were determined to create a welcoming environment where all could comfortably share their challenges and successes. Brian Kennedy ('15) suggested to officially name this growing organization The Physical Therapy Pro Bono Network. He developed a logo for the marketing materials and added a page to the clinic website.

With the growing Physical Therapy Pro Bono Network and the commitment to host annual conferences, the Student Board decided to add a new position: Conference Chair. Nicole Nardone assumed this position for the Class of 2015 followed by Melinda Berean ('16), Nicole Rayson ('17), Jenna Newton ('18), Jon Rouse ('19) and Alaina Curry ('20). Each conference chair and each class added more ideas and further refined the event. Just like the student-run model for the pro bono clinic, this became a student-run model for planning and hosting conferences.

This conference on Widener University's campus continued to grow. By the third year, the Conference Chairs were discussing how to deal with the rapidly expanding interest. The majority of the attendees were coming from the East Coast. Many students within a day's driving distance were piling into cars and driving up or down the interstate to reach Philadelphia. Others were flying in to the nearby Philadelphia airport. For the second and third year of conferences, virtual attendance was possible for those who were too far away to attend in person. Brian Kennedy ('15), Jon Bellizio ('16), Joe Kiehl ('17) and Zach Mease ('17) were instrumental in facilitating the technology.

When the third conference reached record attendance, the conference planners began thinking bigger. The Student Board members had continued to represent the clinic at various conferences throughout the country. They were encountering more and more programs with interest in what they had to share, and they were not just on the East Coast. While virtual attendance was possible, it just did not compare to the energy and experience of attending in person.

I wish to make a side note here. The inspiration that comes from conferences cannot be described in words. It's something that you should add to your recipe for success if you are not already doing so. If you have students who are reluctant to attend conferences, we strongly encourage you to share this book with them. Likewise, I encourage faculty and programs to seek out ways to support student conference attendance and participation. The experience will be transformative for the students, your program, and the future of the profession.

With the evident growth in the third conference and the interest that was coming from beyond the East Coast, the Conference Chairs started to think bigger. Nicole Rayson ('16) and Daria Porretta ('16) approached Jill with great enthusiasm and said, "How about we host a second annual conference on the West Coast?"

Jill was not so enthusiastic. Sometimes the students have such grandiose ideas and they lack the wisdom and practical experience to know that such grandiose ideas are not practical and not possible. She explained to them that this would be a huge undertaking and began to list the seemingly insurmountable barriers. They would need to find a host venue to partner with them. They would need to secure sponsorship of at least $6000 in order to send a cohort of students to the conference to run it. They would need to do twice the amount of work soliciting and vetting proposals, marketing and following-up on registrations, and finding keynote speakers who would go to both conferences and deliver their presentation for free. (All keynote speakers to date have presented *pro bono* with the conference covering only their traveling and hotel expenses.)

Seemingly insurmountable barriers, right?

Well, the students did not consider them to be insurmountable and asked for a chance to make it happen. Nicole and Daria were going to be graduating but they pulled in Melinda Berean ('17) and her class to get involved. This is often how things work with the Student Board. The older members experience things and look back and see how it could be better, but they don't have the opportunity to implement their ideas because they are graduating and moving on. So, they share their ideas with the cohort behind them and that group gets to implement the ideas as well as put their own spin on them.

Melinda and her cohort successfully secured more than $6000 in sponsorship. They found a host partner in Dr. Misha Bradford and her students at the University of Utah in Salt Lake City where they had just launched their own student-run pro bono clinic the year before. Dr. Ira Gorman, President of the Health, Policy and Administration Section, proved to be a compelling keynote speaker who was willing to travel to both conferences and share his thoughts *pro bono*.

Year four officially marked the successful enactment of two Physical Therapy Pro Bono Network Conferences, one on each side of the country.

As this book is going to press, the student leaders from the Class of 2020 have added a third conference for 2019. In addition to the Eastern Conference at Widener and a Western one at the University of Utah, there will be a conference in the Midwest at the Southwestern Baptist University in Bolivar, Missouri.

The clinic was now not only operating in and impacting Chester, but also making waves nationally. Schools from all over the country now had a place to meet to discuss challenges, goals, and ideas, learning from one another and from the many variations of physical therapy pro bono work. Figure 4 depicts the locations of the growing pro bono network.

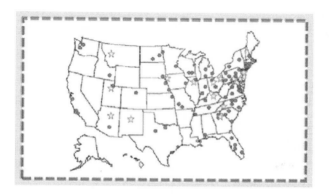

Figure 4. Locations of physical therapy pro bono clinics associated with the growing Pro Bono Network.

Class of 2014 Community Relations Officer, Courtney Christman, posed another grandiose idea: "Let's create a physical therapy pro bono national honor society that would recognize students all over the country that are engaging in pro bono work!" Courtney had experiences in undergraduate honor societies, and she wanted to create something new for pro bono recognition. The Faculty Board did not initially take her seriously, but she persisted in doing the legwork to see her idea forward.

When I first heard about all of this from Courtney, my cell phone almost fell out of my hand! I was so impressed with the repeated innovation of the student leaders and how enthusiastic they were about their peers across the country who shared their same commitment to pro bono service. I asked, "Why would anyone bother to build a National Honor Society?" and Courtney's response was amazing! She stated she was moved by how much work and dedication to the pro bono clinic she saw in her classmates and knew of the work done in the classes before hers to create the clinic. She understood that they accomplished all of this in addition to keeping up with their rigorous academic curriculum, and they did it with such a commitment to provide the best care they could for the community. This was the catalyst that sparked her desire to formally honor these students.

Launching an Honor Society is not easy or intuitive. Courtney worked on this project the entire three years of her DPT curriculum. With pride, she saw it launched in May of 2014 and her class was the first graduating class to have this potential designation. One of the big challenges in creating the guidelines for the honor came with trying to decide how many hours of service merited recognition. Courtney polled all of the programs that came to the conferences and they concluded that each member institution would set their own criteria for recognition. This allowed each institution to have flexibility and ownership in recognizing their star pro bono students. Courtney was thrilled to offer committed students the recognition. She hoped that they would take pride in their work and boldly list the honor on their resume. Since Courtney launched the honor society, the eight inaugural institutional members have grown to twenty-eight! Hundreds of students receive the honor each year. When Courtney graduated, the question became: "How do we sustain the operation of the Honor Society?" Guess how. The Student Board added another position: National Pro Bono Honor Society Officer.

Impact is about what you are doing for others. The conferences, the Honor Society, and the network all aim to have a positive impact on students, faculty, communities, the profession, and the clients. Get involved with The Network! Join the Honor Society. Attend one of the conferences! Your next big idea may come from attending a conference. That is exactly how the most powerful ideas at Widener have started. Put yourself out there and give yourself the best chance to succeed at a high level. Wayne Gretzky may have said it best: "You miss one-hundred percent of the shots you never take." Take your shot. Make it to a conference. If not the ones by Widener on the East and West Coast attend those that the APTA and other organizations have so you can learn from your peers in the field and be set to make positive impacts.

Nothing illustrates impact and success more than seeing the continued involvement someone has after they leave a program. Where there is smoke, there is fire. In parallel, where there is a successful program, there are dedicated alumni. The greatest thing about impacting the lives of the students at the clinic and seeing them succeed after school was their dedication to coming back to the school to help.

A thriving alumni base that continues to give back is one that was positively impacted when they were fully engaged in what the program offered. I, for one, can speak personally on how uninvolved or disengaged I've been with my alma mater. One of the major reasons I have not engaged is because I was not involved much while attending the school.

The student-led model eliminates complacency completely because students are one-hundred percent engaged in their learning experience; in fact, they are creating it! This, I believe, created the bridge for alumni to give back to the school and serve in many different capacities. I spoke to graduates who honestly could not wait to give back even if they moved to another part of the country. Some of the alumni had hired recent graduates and even more were advisors and supervisors, returning to support the current students running the clinic. One alum, Aaron Peffer ('11) moved to Kentucky to follow his girlfriend and sought out an opportunity to be a licensed supervisor in the University of Kentucky's student-run pro bono clinic. Christina Guay ('14) moved near DeSales University and will help their physical therapy pro bono clinic as it launches.

The continued commitment of the alumni is not surprising. They were the same students who had left something for the classes that came after them and did it without expecting credit. They were the ones that invested in the Big Picture and it was the Big Picture that continued to drive them. I remember my conversations with Wayne, and he explained that he moved away to Georgia for a few years but did not move away from his commitment to the clinic. As soon as he relocated closer to school again, he jumped right back in. He said he feels it is something that is expected. The very same open-door policy that was available to him as a student was also there to welcome him back. It was a forgone conclusion that when you could, you would give back. I believe this spirit of service is a result of the community culture that started and sustains the clinic.

If you're going to have a thriving community culture, make sure those in the community have not been forced to be there. This allows both the product and the service to thrive. Those who aren't invested often are the reasons great ships sink. As an unknown wise man or woman once said, "Ships don't sink because of the water around them; ships sink because of the water that gets in them."

The community culture at Widener is one of service from the top down and bottom up. Widener University's webpage states, "… we achieve our mission by creating a learning environment where curricula are connected to societal issues through civic engagement." The Institute for Physical Therapy Education's (IPTE) mission is "to graduate clinically competent physical therapists that demonstrate exemplary character and assume the responsibilities of citizenship." I already shared the mission of the IPTE Center for Community Engagement and the mission of the Chester Community Physical Therapy Clinic. Service is woven throughout this University and created a prime foundation for the clinic project to flourish.

That said, not every Doctor of Physical Therapy (DPT) student arrived at Widener excited to be part of the clinic.

The first few years, only the cohort of students who volunteered to serve on the Student Board volunteered to treat in the clinic. In that first year, the clinic was only open two evenings a week and only had a few clients each night. Occasionally, students not on the Board volunteered and spoke very positively of their experience. More and more students began to volunteer, making the Student Relations Officer's scheduling responsibility easier. In the fall of 2012, Haelim Park joined the Board as the Class of 2015 Student Relations Officer. The Student Relations Officers above her taught her the job responsibilities, which included requesting classmates to volunteer their service.

Haelim questioned how this job was accomplished. Despite the practice of non-mandated service, her feeling was, "This is such a great opportunity for my classmates. Why shouldn't everyone participate?!" She proceeded to schedule ALL of her classmates to serve in the clinic. At first, the Faculty Board was concerned that the students forced to be there would sink the ship. They chose to watch and wait rather than interfere. An amazing thing happened. The first-year Class of 2015 students dutifully reported to their clinic service without complaint.

In reality, the new Class of 2015 didn't realize that previous classes had a choice about serving in the clinic. They made the assumption that this was what was expected, and there was enough positive momentum in the clinic that they just stepped in and added to it. This created a whole NEW culture shift. It was now a part of the Institute of Physical Therapy Education (IPTE) culture at Widener University that all DPT students serve in the clinic. If you don't want to be a part of the pro bono clinic, don't apply to Widener.

Figure 5 depicts the DPT student involvement and the student leadership involvement in the clinic throughout their three-year curriculum.

STUDENT BOARD Involvement through the Three-Year Curriculum

	June	July	Aug	Sept	Oct	Nov	Dec	Jan	Feb	March	April	May
Year 1	Orient	Apply	Named								RUN	RUN
Year 2	RUN	RUN	RUN	RUN		RUN					off	off
Year 3	off	off	off	Senior Schola	Senior Schola	Senior Schola	off	off	off	off	off	

DPT STUDENT Involvement through the Three Year Curriculum

	June	July	Aug	Sept	Oct	Nov	Dec	Jan	Feb	March	April	May
Year 1	Obs.	Obs.	Obs.									
Year 2											off	off
Year 3	off	off	off	Mentor	Mentor	Mentor	off	off	off	off	off	

A similar culture of involvement emerged within the IPTE faculty. As described previously, the Faculty Board initially consisted of Kerstin, Jill, and Robin Dole, leaving seven other faculty members without formal roles or responsibilities in the clinic. The Faculty Board chose not to mandate faculty involvement. Mandating faculty service would have made it a lot easier on the Alumni/ Supervisor Relations Officer, as it was their main responsibility to schedule licensed supervisors for each night. Surprisingly, ALL of the faculty have served as supervisors in the clinic of their own accord. The Alumni/Supervisor Relations Officers often reach out to faculty if the regularly scheduled supervisor is unable to attend on a given night. A faculty member usually steps in to fill the gap. Sometimes faculty show up in the clinic unannounced and speak to the client care that falls within their area of expertise. This practice serves as a win-win for both client care and the student learning experience.

In addition to serving voluntarily as supervisors in the clinic, faculty have found their own individual ways of supporting the students and their efforts in the clinic. We already shared that Dr. Sam Pierce routinely offers his support in the planning of the 5K, and Dr. Dawn Gulick provides expertise in running continuing education courses to raise profits for the clinic. Doctors Bob Wellmon and Sandy Campbell are both skilled photographers, and they routinely respond to the student call to capture events in the clinic or at conferences. These are just some examples of the culture of commitment among the faculty.

The culture of commitment is also very evident in the alumni that return, ready to support the current students and continue to serve the clients as supervisors. In the last nine years, thirty-six alumni have participated as supervisors. The students expressed great appreciation for these alumni. While their textbooks teach them standard techniques, the alumni that have been out practicing bring in a fresh, real-life perspective. The students also appreciate the different perspectives, recognizing that not every clinician does things the same way. The students were learning early on to deal with disparities. Talk about a great learning experience! The students in the clinic are participating in authentic learning experiences that extend way beyond their typical classroom experience.

Another thing that was impressive was seeing former students like Mike McDevitt, who now owns his own clinic, returning to work in the clinic. Mike serves on Thursdays as a supervisor. If he isn't available, he makes sure one of his employees is able to cover. In other words, Mike's company commits to filling the secondary supervisor need on Thursday nights.

The clinic has positions for Primary and Secondary Supervisors. The Institute for Physical Therapy hires and pays primary supervisors as adjunct faculty members. Primary supervisors commit to a consistent night each week, providing consistency for both students and clients. In the early years, only one supervisor was present per night, but as the clinic got busier, the Student and Faculty Board enlisted two supervisors a night and moved to paying primary supervisors to improve consistency. Supervisors receive the adjunct hourly lab instructor rate. Secondary supervisors invest in volunteering on a less consistent basis, perhaps monthly or weekly.

Here's the schedule for a typical licensed supervisor such as Mike. See Figure 6. Client care starts at 4:30 pm, so Mike and the students arrive between 4:00 and 4:10 pm to go over the client charts. The treating student and supervisor have a conversation about the plan for each client. Mike answers any questions and allows the students to work through proposed plans. Once clients start to arrive, the student therapists take the lead and Mike guides and directs as needed.

Sample Schedule

Pre-PT Receptionist	Melissa				
Licensed Supervisors	Wayne & Christine				
Student Clinic Administrator	Georgia (PTIII), Joe (PTI)				
Student Therapists	Team A: Alanna (PTIII), Kyle(PTII), Nolan (PTI)		Team B: Brian(PTIII), Daria (PTII), Maggie(PTI)		Team C: Nicole(PTIII), Nicole R (PTII), Lauren PTI
4:30	Team A Client	Team A Client	Team B Client	Team B Client	Team C Client	Team C Client
5:30	Team A Client		Team B Client		Team C Client	Team C Client

Figure 6. Sample Schedule

Clients arrive at 4:30 and 5:30 pm. The 5:30 clients typically finish up at 6:30 pm and the student therapists move into documenting their treatment sessions. As discussed previously, the students document with WebPT and use iPads or their own mobile devices. Supervisors provide guidance as needed. When the students complete their patient notes, they forward them for finalization by the licensed supervisor. This gives the supervisor an opportunity to go over the notes with the student in detail, making any corrections or suggestions before signing off on the note. In this way, the students get practice in real-world documentation prior to their first full-time clinical experiences.

When it comes to community culture at the clinic, it is very clear that pride and professionalism exudes from everyone from top to bottom. If the definition of culture is the way of doing things, then the culture produced within the Institute for Physical Therapy Education is one that many others would like to implement and see continued in the physical therapy profession.

Scott Voshell exemplifies this pride and professionalism. He was a part of the initial advisory committee to the Institute for Physical Therapy Education about twenty-three years ago. When the clinic was launched in 2009, he became one of the first members of the clinic's Advisory Board. The culture of giving students a first-hand experience impressed him so much that he hired students to work as part of his organization at Main Line Health where he served as the Director of Rehabilitation. When I asked him the reason he employs students who have served at the pro bono clinic, his response was that the students simply have an upper hand coming from this program compared to others. They have the best teacher anyone can ask for—firsthand experience—from the very beginning of the curriculum. Scott himself is an excellent role model for the students, serving the physical therapy profession through leadership in the state professional organization.

So, what can we gather from the idea of building a community culture of commitment, pride, and professionalism? The culture creates a pipeline that ensures the best level of instruction and expertise is always available. Mentoring is a huge component of someone's success, and building a culture centered on giving back, contributing to those that come after, and staying connected are big contributors to culture.

When building a community culture there are some keys that cannot be overlooked. One, you must have a welcoming environment for those who leave your program and want to come back and help in any way they can. The best organizations have a rich history of people coming back and shaping the future generations. Take the New York Yankees, for example. No team in baseball has won more championships than the New York Yankees. It's also no coincidence that no team has a tradition quite like the Yankees. Examples of tradition that build the culture include their vintage pinstripes; old-timer games where past players take the field; and spring training when old-timers returning attend and mentor the current players. Once a Yankee, always a Yankee. All Yankees, including the players, the fans, and the organization, benefit.

Any organization can benefit from having strong mentor relationships. For an organization to thrive, mentoring should be a part of your organizational growth plan. The positive culture and firsthand feedback that mentors share with students will serve them now and in their future careers.

I want to mention something that, at first, I found surprising, and then I realized is part of the success of the culture. Students address their faculty by their first name, not by a title and last names. I learned from Dr. Robin Dole that this custom has been in place since the Institute for Physical Therapy Education started twenty-three years ago. I wondered "Why?" Is it because they wanted to appear informal? To make the environment more chill or relaxed? It was neither. Robin explained that the reason for this practice was because the faculty consider themselves future colleagues of the students and expect the students to respect them without the formality of a title, as you would respect a colleague. When I heard this, I felt like someone was telling me the secret recipe for Kentucky Fried Chicken or something. It's often funny, isn't it, how the simplest things work so well? It's not a revolutionary thought; however, it was one that has a tremendous impact on the culture between students and faculty. To go and speak to Jill Black and say, "Hey, Jill, I have an idea" was a lot easier and welcoming than to say, "Dr. Black, I have an idea." The difference is subtle but was significant to the students. They told me repeatedly that they valued the relationship. They said things such as, "It meant that they were one of us, that there was no difference in class. We are all at the same level." This is also called future pacing. Future pacing is where you speak to people as if they were at a future place in time. Sure, the students had not even finished their coursework, but they were already being treated as if they had.

It is quite obvious now why students come back, right? It is clear why students would graduate and crave giving back to the clinic, even if it's occasionally taking on the role of a licensed supervisor or running in the 5K. It's the culture of commitment that is clearly established.

CHAPTER 9:
SPACE EXPANSION

Are you familiar with Shark Tank? Not a literal tank with sharks, but the ABC television show. The show features top entrepreneurs such as the owner of the NBA Dallas Mavericks Mark Cuban and Real Estate Mogul Barbara Corcoran, just to name a few. These entrepreneurs listen as aspiring tycoons make pitches to sell a portion of their business to them. I'm a huge fan of the show because I love the art of pitching an idea. When one makes a pitch, the job is to present the idea, reveal the product's sales figures, and identify what is wanted from the entrepreneur "sharks" of the show. The worst pitches are the ones that ignore key principles that make for an effective pitch such as, "Is there a need in the marketplace?" And, "What are the potential barriers and how will you overcome them?"

You might be asking, "What does this have to do with a student-led pro bono physical therapy clinic in Chester, PA?" Great question. As I learned about the efforts of the Student Board to make pitches for new space, I realized there was a parallel between what they were doing and Shark Tank. Students would have to craft and present a proposal for more space. This is not an easy task. Space is something that is limited everywhere. With limited supply and sometimes-unlimited demand, it is quite the challenge to acquire new or additional space.

As I interviewed the student leaders that served across a span of eight years, I realized that "we needed more space" was a frequent refrain, because of the consistent and dramatic clinic growth. Remember the humble beginnings of one two-month old client that first week? Well, a second client was added the second week, and more and more after that! The clinic growth was slow in the beginning, but the Faculty Board was not concerned. They wanted the students to get things in place and to have opportunities to "get it right" on a small scale before treating the masses. This is a lesson to remember if an idea does not appear to be a huge hit right out the gate. A good idea warrants a sustained effort to ensure that it's potential can be realized. Putting forth such an effort is exactly what the program at Widener did. They stuck with it and as they had small successes, they increased their marketing efforts to allow for more growth. As community relations improved and marketing efforts advanced, more and more clients began to come.

Within four months, the clinic went from two evenings a week to three. Within a year, it was open four. By the third year, the need was exceeding the 700 square foot space that was available. Hours could not be extended because of the students' class schedules. This growth was both a great experience and a great challenge for the students. They were asking themselves, "How can we possibly provide the same high-quality care that we did from the start when we have only so much space for students and clients?" Schedules were getting packed as more clients were coming, and the students were reluctant to create a waiting list.

The students couldn't expand hours, but they certainly could schedule more students and more supervisors within the hours they had IF they had more space. They began to explore their space options. As I said earlier, they were sharing this old home with the Neuropsychological Assessment Center (NAC). NAC was using their space in the day; the clinic was using its space in the evening. What if they sought dual purpose options for the space? This was a tricky proposition because it entailed moving into NAC space and asking them to share it.

The students expressed to me that they did not want to step on the toes of another department and make one department's space needs more important than another's. This courtesy is something that easily could have been missed or overlooked by so many. Too many times we might be so caught up in our own priorities that we do not think about how we may be affecting others. The students worked to see how they could create a common office the physical therapy clinic could share with NAC, improving upon their office space and seeking a win-win. This was quite the challenge, to say the least, but once again the students—motivated by solutions and not egos—were able to find a compromise where all stakeholders would be content.

The plans for the dual-purposing of space happened under Scott Cheney's ('13 Clinic Coordinator) watch. The 2013 Operations Coordinators Kate Conahan and Lauren Papps had already overseen a space makeover of the basement that was now used for storage. They were the ones who posed the ideas for dual-purposing space on the first floor of the home. Class of 2014 Operations Coordinator, Jake Daniels, carried their ideas forward, negotiated the deal, and saw the space expansion happen. Once completed, the additional space allowed the clinic to see double the clientele. The space expansion involved collaboration and cooperation with the Neuropsychological Assessment Center (NAC). Prior, this space was separate. The new space was built to facilitate dual purpose as parts could be used by the NAC by day and the clinic in the evenings.

For those reading this, it is important to remember that when you are pitching anything, you want to have a win-win relationship. This is something that is spoken about in the best-selling book *7 Habits of Highly Effective People*, by Stephen R. Covey. The book talks about seeking win-win relationships, not for the sake of being nice or to have a quick-fix but instead as a great mode for maximum human interaction and collaboration—two cornerstones of the clinic.

Let's stay on the topic of space for a moment. You'll read in a later chapter how the clinic begins to grow inter-professionally. With this inter-professional incorporation of service came a need for … you guessed it … more space.

The faculty and student leaders knew that they had reached the full space potential at their current site. To expand further would require moving to a new and bigger site. With space at a premium across the university, such a move would be a lot harder to negotiate than the previous space expansion. Desiring to start somewhere, Jill charged the Class of 2017 Operations Coordinators to design a dream space and develop a proposal to sell it. She did this as part of their third-year clinic project assignment associated with PT775, one of their final DPT classes. Joe Kiehl and Zach Mease eagerly accepted the challenge.

Like a good Shark Tank proposal, Joe and Zach set out to clearly articulate the need. They identified that an overcrowded clinic was a problem because it could cause anxiety for the clients (and students!), compromise confidentiality, and create safety hazards such as tripping over one another. All of these concerns might sound extreme, but they certainly were warranted on busy nights … and most nights were now busy.

Joe and Zach took pictures of the space on crowded nights to document the need. They captured student therapists performing functional walk tests out in the parking lot because there wasn't enough room inside the clinic. Zach completed an ADA assessment checklist and pointed out where the current space was non-compliant.

Not only did they identify how the clinic's space was inadequate and out of compliance, but they proposed a completely new dream space as part of their project. Joe's brother was a professional architect and willingly volunteered his time and skill to create an architectural drawing of the students' vision. The students had the footprint dimensions of an old, vacant middle school building on the edge of campus. They created a dream inter-professional space that could fill the first floor of the 150 x 250 square foot footprint.

The students knew that simply describing the space problem would not drive change; they also needed to paint a vision of the future clinic. This vision included adding more interdisciplinary health fields to the clinic. In the beginning, the clinic was only for physical therapy but adding other disciplines such as psychology and occupational therapy would create a unique model. The faculty was thrilled to see how this multi-dimensional proposal was progressing.

As part of the project assignment, Jill required them to actually deliver the proposal to someone. She asked if Robin Dole (Associate Dean and Program Director) and Paula Silver (Dean of the School of Human Service Professions) would be willing to be an audience. Both Associate Dean Dole and Dean Silver agreed and gave an hour of their time to listen to the student space proposal.

Joe and Zach were ready and passionate about their topic! Their passion came through and by the time they concluded with the architectural drawing, Dean Silver applauded and then asked, "Do you know about the new capital campaign initiative? I think this would be perfect to pitch for that."

Unbeknownst to the students or the faculty, Widener University was preparing to embark on a new capital campaign and would be soliciting proposals for what they were calling "The Big Idea." The Big Idea was to be something transformative, inter-professional, and in alignment with the university mission. Wow! Joe and Zach's proposal met all of the criteria. Unfortunately, they were getting ready to move into their final clinical rotations and would be off campus until they returned for graduation in May. They knew what to do. It is what they always do. Pass their good ideas on to the leaders behind them.

In Silicon Valley, proposals or pitches are made daily. Someone, right now as you are reading this book, is probably working on a pitch deck asking for more space, more funding, more support, more something! Zach and Joe and the students that followed felt the process of having to make a proposal was challenging and rewarding.

They took their proposal to Tim Golder ('18 Clinic Coordinator), Steve Grazioli ('18 Health and Wellness Coordinator), and Seth Brakefield ('18 Operations Coordinator), who eagerly embraced it and added to it. Within a month, they had an opportunity to present it to a larger audience of inter-professional faculty members. They attended meetings where they learned how to best write the proposal for university review. They worked with faculty to help prepare it for submission that spring, with the hope that the university would recognize their idea as the most feasible and best Big Idea. With university and donor backing, their student-run physical therapy pro bono clinic could become a student-run inter-professional pro bono clinic fantastic for the clients, fantastic for the students growing in inter-professional skills, and fantastic for the university.

Just months ago, they learned that their idea is the top choice among more than sixty submissions, and that the university is actively seeking donors for this project. As I write this book, the Big Idea proposal has been passed down to Reed Hofmann ('19 Operations Coordinator) and Justin Gilfillan ('19 Clinic Coordinator). The hope is that one day, all of the student leaders will be able to come back for the ribbon cutting of the new space they had imagined.

As the reader, what you can take away from this account is how much of a process it really is to create and sell a Big Idea. Momentum is critical to advance big ideas. If you currently have nothing, then start something. The clinic was able to make a proposal with confidence as a result of their clinic's impact, and the contributions of returning students. Collaborating with others to make a big idea better, and not just focusing on your needs, is a reliable lesson, but one that is not always easy to follow. Many times, egos can get in the way of great accomplishments, because claiming credit takes precedence over collaborating.

Together Everyone Achieves More (TEAM) is a classic mantra of a team approach.

The truth of this saying is perfectly illustrated in the inter-professional clinic proposal, which, when funded, will immeasurably enrich Widener students and the broader community. Pretty powerful stuff, if you ask me.

CHAPTER 10:
GRAND ROUNDS

There I was, sitting there in deep thought, complaining in my head about what should be or could be done. Have you ever had that moment? A moment where you've been making some observations and realized that all was not great, and something needed to be improved? Did you do anything about it or keep the thoughts to yourself? There have been many instances where a suggestion could have helped someone or improved a situation, and I "let the cat get my tongue" as the expression says. My reaction was, "I hope they will figure it out" or "I hope things just get better." This approach signifies a reactive mindset, not a proactive one

Earlier I mentioned the book *7 Habits of Highly Effective People* by Stephen R. Covey and the habit of creating win-win situations. In that book, he also details the habit of being proactive. In fact, this habit is so important that is the first of the seven.

Being proactive is not waiting for something to fall apart before taking action. There is a quote by John F. Kennedy I love which states, "The best time to repair a roof is when the sun is shining." This is obviously easier said than done but is the mark of a well-functioning organization or human being.

At the clinic, students began to notice that as the client numbers were growing and the entire student body was providing care (remember Haelim Park started the trend to schedule everybody?), consistency in client care was suffering and students were feeling ill-prepared to work with their clients. Sometimes when you grow at a rapid pace, things can be missed or easily overlooked. It's like the sports adage that says, "Winning covers it all." Sometimes you can be winning so much that you do not take the time to see how there are areas of improvements that you could still make to get even better. The students did not feel this way. They constantly kept what Carol Dweck calls a "growth mindset." They were practicing what my friend likes to call "Kaizen," which is the mindset of always improving.

This is how the idea of the Grand Rounds began. It was in 2015--when the clinic had been continuing to grow year after year, developing a positive reputation, and meeting client needs-- that students started to think, "How can we better handle the growing numbers? What is it that we can do to take our clinic to the next level? How may we better serve our clients? How can we help students to be more prepared for treating the many clients in the clinic?" It was these questions that helped drive the conversation of creating something where students would be able to meet together and discuss client care.

At the time, 150 students were actively involved in the clinic. It's no surprise that with that many students, things could be missed. Hence, the Class of 2015 posed an idea: Why not divide the active clients into three teams, and divide the student body into three teams as well? This would improve the chances that clients and students would get to know one another, building better rapport and confidence. In addition to forming teams, the student leaders began adding a weekly "Grand Rounds" class into the curriculum. In Grand Rounds, the students would meet and discuss the client cases on their team.

Let me pause a minute and visit this thought about the clinic and connections to the curriculum. When the clinic started, not every student was serving in the clinic, only the student leaders were. The student leaders signed up for a "class" that was created specifically to link the clinic to the curriculum. In this way, the university liability policy covered them in the clinic. As for the volunteering supervisors, they needed to purchase an individual malpractice policy; if they were volunteering regularly, the clinic fund would cover the cost.

In the beginning, a few professors allowed the students to serve in the clinic in lieu of an assignment. Sometimes class assignments could be completed in the clinic. As these practices grew, the faculty added a statement to all of the course syllabi that stated: "Students enrolled in a course in the entry-level DPT curriculum may be required or elect to gain additional exposure and experience to the content of required and elective courses by participating in the Chester Community Pro Bono Clinic as an extension of the learning activities of the course." In this way, students were covered by the blanket liability and malpractice policies of the university and program.

Once Haelim Park came along and started scheduling all the students in the clinic, the faculty had the opportunity to further connect assignments to the clinic experience. A kinesiology palpation assignment needed to be completed on a real client under the supervision of one of the licensed supervisors or a third-year mentor. Blood pressure check-offs started occurring in the clinic. Documentation assignments connected to the authentic setting of the clinic. Reflections about diversity and social determinants of health arose out of experiences at the clinic. Even teaching and learning and mentorship reflections about experiences in the clinic became a relevant requirement.

Dr. Sandy Campbell, who teaches management and administration, allows the Student Board to complete her Policy and Procedure assignment with the creation or enhancement of a clinic policy and procedure. Faculty and students are continuing to find ways to connect the classroom to the authentic learning experience of the pro bono clinic.

Just to clarify, all of the DPT students spend time treating in the clinic under the Physical Therapist licensed supervisors that come in each night. Anytime that students are on campus and not off on a full-time clinical, they are scheduled to be in the clinic. They do not get specific class credit for this time, but faculty do link assignments to the clinic as noted previously. The student leaders who comprise the Student Board are about 1/5 of a class of students. The other 4/5s of the students participate in one of four after-school activity programs happening out in the community. Both the Student Board members and the Community Activity Program students take a one-credit course for the five semesters that they are on campus.

In this way, the Student Board members are accountable for what they do in service to the clinic. The five-credit sequence of DPT courses is PT771, PT772, PT773, PT774, and PT775. We call it "Community Health Practicum." As students progress through the practicum, they become increasingly responsible for providing mentorship and conducting assessments and evaluations on the success of their respective programs. The space proposal that you read about earlier is an example of how a project fulfilled a course requirement while also advancing the clinic.

One other DPT course that has direct links to clinic projects is PT818: Health Promotion and Wellness. PT818 is a weeklong course that occurs in late spring of the first year. At this point, the third-year students are graduating, and the second-year students are out on a full-time clinical education experience. The first-year students are now the only force in the clinic, and it will be that way for the summer months. In PT818, one of the requirements of the Student Board members is to identify a challenge in the clinic and pose a potential solution. Students then develop a related intervention and seek to pilot that intervention for the next four to six months. They are responsible for measuring outcomes along the way and at the end they present a full evaluation of their pilot.

This assignment has become a means of trialing solutions before completely implementing them. Sometimes the pilot does not work, as in the case of a recent incentive program designed to reduce the cancel and no-show rate. When a pilot completely fails, the pilot changes do not become permanent. Other times the pilot partially works, but students are able to make recommendations for how to design it better the next time. Measuring client clinical outcomes is a good example of this.

For the last three years, a group of students have been working on refining ways of tracking client clinical outcomes. Nolan Converse ('17 Clinic Coordinator) and Kyle Hughes ('17 Outcomes Coordinator) made the first attempt at tracking client clinical outcomes in a meaningful way. At the end of the six months, they found that they had been using too many different outcome tools and did not have a large enough sample size to be able to draw significant conclusions. They then passed their project on to Tim Golder ('18 Clinic Coordinator) and Tyler Suruskie ('18 Outcomes Coordinator).

Tim and Tyler designed their pilot with just two outcome-tracking tools and while they had less diversity across tools, the mechanisms they had in place to ensure that all clients were tracked with these tools did not work. They passed their project on to Taylor Stone ('19 Outcomes Coordinator).

Taylor had time on her hands due to an unexpected medical challenge, and she chose to expand this client clinical outcome project to include four other institutions with student-run pro bono clinics. This multi-institution project has received Institutional Review Board approval and is underway at the time of the writing of this book.

Let's go back to the Class of 2015's Teams and Grand Rounds idea. The Class of 2015 was getting ready to move off to the final full-time clinical education experience, so they passed the idea down to the Class of 2016. Georgia Spano ('16 Health and Wellness Coordinator), Kyle Bauer, ('16 Health and Wellness Coordinator), Sarah Voelkel ('16 Alumni/Supervisor Relations Officer), and Kerry McIntyre (Class of 2016) picked up the project for their PT818 assignment.

They divided their classmates into three teams and the clients into corresponding teams. Each team of students would meet every third Wednesday over lunch to discuss the client cases. Team A one week, Team B the next, Team C the third week, and then the cycle would repeat. One of the clinic supervisors volunteered to provide oversight and guidance for all of the team meetings. The purpose of the meetings was for students to discuss client care, identify ways to progress the program, discuss discharge plans, and increase awareness from one student to the next so that the student therapist would be more familiar with the client and the plan of care.

The six-month pilot proved to be a success with students and clients; supervisors noted improvement in rapport, continuity of care, and progression of the client programs. Grand Rounds fostered additional community building as students and faculty together met with the intent of continuing to provide high quality care consistently. The students went to the faculty and requested that Grand Rounds be added to the curriculum. The faculty honored the request.

Grand Rounds continued to run every fall, spring, and summer semester, and occurred every three weeks for each team until the Class of 2019 came and said, "Can we meet more often?" They felt that reviewing their clients' cases every three weeks was not enough and wanted more. Faculty added another willing supervisor, Mike McDevitt, to the Grand Rounds class, and the student teams started meeting every other week. When all three classes are on campus, the third-year students provide mentorship to the first- and second-year students in the team meeting. First-year students are expected to report out on the basic client information while second-year students are expected to pose program-progressing ideas.

Professor Mark Paterson is a newer addition to the Widener Institute for Physical Therapy Education faculty and has a keen interest and expertise in leading case conferences. He has jumped on the opportunity to help provide guidance in Grand Rounds, and often volunteers in the clinic as needed. Mark has brought new ideas to the structure of reporting in Grand Rounds and has worked collaboratively with the students to implement them.

The addition of Grand Rounds did not completely solve the client continuity challenge, though. The Class of 2019 is currently piloting a "Client Liaison Project," or otherwise known as the "Primary Student Therapist Project" to see if that will help further improve things. The Primary Student Physical Therapist has the job of tracking the client through their entire episode of care. While not involved in every treatment session, the Primary Student Physical Therapist maintains communication with the client, shares progress in Grand Rounds, and leads program progression and discharge planning for the client. Stay tuned for the results of these pilots!

For you who are reading this, be proactive by routinely assessing how things are going within your organizations, your programs, or even with yourself. This awareness provides feedback so you can continue not only to grow but in a sustainable way. One of the benefits inherent in the student-run model is that you have fresh eyes and perspectives coming into leadership every year. We too can benefit by taking fresh looks and by creating forums for open and creative discussion. Strive to be proactive. Do not wait until all things fall apart before doing something. It is a habit that highly effective people use, and one that Widener students are implementing to stay ahead of the curve.

CHAPTER 11:
ADDING SERVICES

Tell me what the following pairs of people have in common:

+ Run DMC and Aerosmith

+ Boyz II Men and Mariah Carey

+ Michael Jackson and Quincy Jones

+ Wilbur and Orville Wright

+ Larry Page and Sergey Brin

If you answered, "These are all famous collaborations," then you would be right. Run DMC and Aerosmith together had the classic "Walk This Way," while Boyz II Men and Mariah Carey sang the popular song "One Sweet Day," and Michael Jackson and Quincy Jones came together to create "Thriller." All within the music industry, these pairs were able to create classics by collaboration. Larry Page and Sergey Brin came together when Brin, a student at Stanford at the time, gave a campus tour to Page. The two would later start the company we know today as Google. Last but not least, we have Wilbur and Orville Wright, also known as the Wright Brothers. You're able to fly around the world because these two great minds came together and developed a flying aircraft after starting out fixing bicycles.

All of these pairs were able to bring something to the world that they most likely would not have been able to without coming together and working with one another.

A similar collaboration took place between Widener University's physical therapy students and Philadelphia University's occupational therapy students. This collaboration arose from the golden formula that has led to many of the clinic innovations—an opportunity and a need.

In the summer of 2015, Nolan Converse ('17 Clinic Coordinator) connected with an occupational therapy (OT) program in the Philadelphia region. He found them to be open to collaboration in the student-run pro bono clinic and asked the Faculty Board if he could invite them to visit the clinic to explore the possibilities. The OT faculty came and met with the PT Faculty Board and it was a match!

Next, Nolan took a presentation to the OT students to explore their interest in adopting the student-run model. He did not want to force this collaboration if there was not buy-in from the students; but the OT students were excited to assume leadership. By January of 2016, the OT students were serving one night per week in the clinic and participating in Grand Rounds every Wednesday afternoon. By Fall of 2016, they had reached their patient capacity leading them to expand their services to two nights per week.

So, what did the program look like, and was there any resistance? One of the challenges—or at least what was perceived to be a problem—was the fact that the program was a weekend hybrid program. The students that Dr. Wendy Wachter-Schutz (OT Faculty member) was responsible for were only local for eight weekends and returned home—usually out of state—during the week. The OT faculty were doubtful that the OT students would be available to work in the clinic on Wednesday evenings. To their amazement, the students gave no pushback and they had no trouble staffing the pro bono clinic.

This commitment clearly showed there was great interest by all stakeholders to make this program successful. What we had was a true interprofessional collaboration, which was beneficial for the students' learning and the community, because now the community members had access to physical therapy and occupational therapy services.

As part of the collaboration with Philadelphia University, the Widener faculty received a grant that required them to collect data on student outcomes. The faculty interviewed licensed OT pro bono clinic supervisors and asked them to share their perceptions about pro bono clinic service, and student preparation for their full-time clinical affiliation. The faculty also surveyed student opinion for full-time clinic readiness both pre- and post- their time at the pro bono clinic.

The data, presented at both Pennsylvania and New Jersey State Occupational Therapy Association conferences in 2018, clearly showed that the OT students had increased confidence and increased clinical reasoning skills after working in the pro bono clinic. They also increased their ability to mentor and be leaders as well. First-year students and second-year students worked together. The second-year students performed the treatment with supervision from the licensed OT and mentored the first-year students. They say if you cannot teach it, then you don't really know it. The pro bono clinic provided the students with an opportunity to show and explain what they learned and what they did.

What also made the PT/OT collaboration special was the leadership. As a student-led pro-bono clinic, the faculty were once again just advisors. There were also student leaders in place that helped with sorting the scheduling, policies, and procedures. At the time of this book being written, Wendy shared that nine of the thirty-five students were clinic student leaders. This gave them an opportunity to run a clinic, schedule patients, find patients, and market the services. These are all cool things that the students normally would not be exposed to in a regular academic program.

This is why this collaboration was so helpful and so exciting. The students were able to not only learn by studying, but also by doing. When supervisors were interviewed, they mentioned that the students came from this program and worked in their facilities were light years ahead of traditional students. Their interviewing and clinical reasoning skills were top notch. Additionally, their experience with electronic documentation placed them ahead of the pack compared to other students. Students with clinic experience were already proficient in skills that would normally be taught during the first few weeks of a paid job. This head start would help jump-start their careers.

There aren't enough words to describe how amazing the pro bono real-life experiences are for the students.

Additional Collaborations

The addition of OT services was not the only service added at this time. Widener University has an Institute for Graduate Clinical Psychology and faculty member Dr. Bret Boyer approached the clinic leadership about the possibility of assigning a graduate clinical psychology doctoral student to the clinic. His vision was that his student would be on the clinic floor all hours of operation, identifying clients who might benefit from clinical psychology services, and either intervening directly on the floor or inviting clients to participate in outpatient counseling services.

At first, the leadership was skeptical to add even one more person because there is so little room in the clinic. And it was unclear to them exactly what the graduate clinical psychology student would be doing with clients in the clinic. But everyone came to an agreement to enact a pilot trial for one year. Scott Thein, doctoral graduate clinical psychology and masters of business administration student, took on the pilot challenge. Scott proceeded to immerse himself in clinic operations and worked with the PT student leadership to determine how to best incorporate his services.

After just one month, it was apparent to all that his services were highly beneficial and that this one-year trial was going to be a huge success. Why? Well, because believe it or not, many of the clients coming to the clinic for physical challenges also had emotional and mental health challenges that Scott was able to help address. In short order, he had more work than he could handle and his recommendation at the conclusion of the pilot was that at least TWO graduate clinical psychology students should be assigned to clinic service next year.

Katie Lawless and Aubrey Flanigan stepped in for year two and did a great job advancing the service that Scott had started. They submitted the following report after just two months of service:

> Our role, as Clinical Psychology students, in the Physical Therapy clinic is founded on the idea of interdisciplinary collaboration. We work together with the physical therapists, occupational therapists, students and patients in order to gain a deeper understanding of the patients' functioning and quality of life. We believe that physical and mental health are deeply intertwined.
>
> In the clinic, we provide brief anxiety, depression, and pain assessments to each incoming patient. With these results, in conjunction with talking to the physical and occupational therapists, we gain a better understanding of who may initially need psychological intervention. In addition to screening patients, we provide both on the floor psychological treatment and outpatient psychotherapy sessions. Both of these services are to help manage psychological factors that may be impeding a patient's ability to adhere to treatment, both in the clinic and at home.
>
> We currently have five regular outpatient clients, three clients that will be potentially beginning outpatient services, and ten patients we regularly check in with,

and work with on the floor, during PT and OT sessions. These numbers continue to grow. We have collaborated with each PT and OT to discuss patients and gain a better understanding of their physical health, while also educating the PTs and OTs on how the patients' psychological functioning is playing a role in their progress.

Together in this collaboration, we have already begun to see the growth in ourselves, PTs, OTs, and clients in gaining a full understanding of every client. This interdisciplinary approach ensures that the client is getting the best practice, while also having all services in one building for easy access. We look forward to continuing this teamwork and are excited to see the growth the clinic continues to make!

The physical therapy students corroborate the benefit that the graduate clinical psychology students bring to the clinic. They see the positive impact that they are having on clients. They appreciate the input they bring to Grand Rounds. They articulate how they are learning more about considering the clients' needs in a more holistic manner.

The graduate clinical psychology interns have helped bring additional health and wellness services to the clinic. They fostered the clinic's relationship with Widener University's Neuropsychological Assessment Center (NAC), making referrals for Neuropsychological testing when necessary. They also welcome a graduate intern from Widener University's Biofeedback Clinic. Tim Overton came to the clinic several times and offered a free trial of biofeedback. The physical therapy students identified several PT clients with stress and cervical dysfunction as potential beneficiaries. Those that trialed it and liked it were offered a series of biofeedback sessions at a significantly reduced rate. The clinic plans to continue this relationship with the Biofeedback Clinic in the coming years.

Widener University also has a Community Nursing Clinic housed within a local non-profit organization called Cityteam Ministries and students have learned to recommend referral to nursing when warranted.

The newest service joining the clinic is Social Work. Widener University's Center for Social Work operates several different community clinics, but the Chester Community Physical Therapy Clinic had never connected with them until 2018. Now, a graduate social work student attends weekly Grand Rounds to hear about each of the client cases and readily offers recommendation on community resources that might be available for the client. The clinic is looking forward to this relationship and the benefits that are bound to come.

The theme of this chapter is that there is great power in collaboration and one of the best ways to find a great collaborating partner is to identify what is missing and find someone who is already doing what you need. Widener did that when Nolan reached out to a neighboring occupational therapy program to pursue a collaboration that would benefit all stakeholders. Dr. Bret Boyer did that when he presented the opportunity for his graduate clinical psychology students to intern in the clinic which has led to the integration of NAC, the Biofeedback Clinic, and now Social Work.

Remember, there were Michael Jackson and Quincy Jones, the Wright Brothers, and now inter-professional services in the student-run pro bono clinic. What collaboration can you envision putting together?

CHAPTER 12:
WIDENER'S EXPERIENCE IN THE COMMUNITY

At this point, you know how the idea of the student-run pro bono clinic at Widener emerged, the model they've used to run it, and the leadership style the faculty used that allowed students to thrive. You've learned how the students had a spirit of "Kaizen" where they always wanted to make improvements for the community good. From putting together a pro bono conference for physical therapy programs, to growing regional conferences, to creating a pro bono national honor society to creating client liaison programs and space proposals, these students have done quite a bit over time. The one thing we have not yet heard are specific stories of the clients served. We've heard how the student-led model was great for the students and how the faculty interacted with the program, but what about the clients?

What was the clinic like from a client's point of view? Kerstin Palombaro provided some insight. She started by explaining that many times clients will max out their insurance before they have gotten one-hundred percent better. Hearing this was very disappointing. It's like having a file download up to ninety percent and never finishing. You never get to enjoy it fully because you never received what you needed completely.

Kerstin then shared with me the story of a client who came to the clinic. She later revealed that the client was actually her younger brother who is an elite marathoner. He had a hip injury for which he was receiving physical therapy treatment elsewhere until he reached his lifetime insurance cap. He came to the pro bono clinic with Kerstin's encouragement. At first, he was skeptical, but he went and later told his sister over and over again how impressed he was with the care that the students gave him. He told her that he thought the care he received from the pro bono clinic was actually better than the treatment he received from traditional clinics. That's right, the students did that. Sounding like a broken record, he continued to sing the praises of the students, from how much they knew to how caring and concerned they were.

This became the new normal for the clinic. Time and time again, the clients will say how much they felt valued, that they were getting better, and that they were not being told they cannot come anymore because of insurance. It is one thing to be told the treatment is not working; but to be getting better and then not able to continue because of financial or insurance reasons is devastating. The pro bono clinic provides that safety net. No longer was the clients' economic status the determining factor of reaching full recovery. Here are a few more quotes from clients about their experience at the Chester Community Physical Therapy Clinic.

> *"I was impressed the first time I came in by everyone here from the sessions to everyone. There is an obvious feeling of compassion. There's no superficial... nobody's superficial here."*

> *"And they aren't afraid to work me at all... at the same time they are very sensitive and will back it down if needed."*

> *"I came in not walking, now I am walking... I would definitely come back."*

> *"They've helped me in every way. I think they are the best."*

Thanks to the clinic providing the services and opportunities, community members are able to move toward healing. This is what leading by needs is all about. In an era when many young people are only focused on themselves, it's impressive and refreshing to see a community of students who are dedicated to giving back to their community and making the well-being of others their highest priority. The students at the clinic understood

Martin Luther King Jr.'s quote: "Life's most urgent and pertinent question is 'What are you doing for others?'" The special students of the clinic absolutely showed me first hand that they aim to live a meaningful life by investing in meaningful work.

I remember every single interview I did with the students, how they were so proud to be involved in impacting their community. Some never considered having any civic duty prior to being plugged into the clinic itself. The clinic provided the path for them to be able to do for others. It's how everything the clinic has done has come together.

This is the kind of work in which legacies are made. These are the things that create memories that last forever and bring smiles to the faces of those who provided the care, and those that benefited. It's this kind of work that drives the student leaders of the clinic to move forward. It's what brought the inspiration to have this story told so that others can see that this idea is bigger than just a clinic. It is about students leading the way to serving the needs of others while learning how to be the best they can be within their profession. It's about faculty that put ego aside for the greater good of the Chester community and Widener students.

An inspiration to say the least, but it does not stop here. With this information, what are you inspired to do in the future that will leave an impact on an entire community? The stories in the book are about real people like you; these stories can also be yours. I hope you're ready—there are people waiting for you to rise up and help them rise up.

CHAPTER 13:
THE STUDENT'S POINT OF VIEW

Have you ever thought something was one way, only to find out it was another?

There's a saying that goes like this: "If you want to know, go to the source".

When it comes to the clinic and how impactful it was on the students, I did just that. I went to the source and asked them one question specifically as I finished all my interviews. The question was: "How did the work you did with the clinic have an impact on your career as a Physical Therapist?" The answers were all different, but the theme was the same. The students felt confident, prepared, and filled with gratitude for the pro bono clinic opportunity. I wanted to share their words exactly so you can get a chance to hear what I heard.

Courtney Christman: (Class of 2014)

The clinic honestly gave me a ton of leadership skills, which I've definitely used at my current job. The things that I've learned from the clinic about what it takes to work as a team, and to really collaborate with other people, has been hugely helpful as there's all different sides to different situations, and to be able to work through them as a team and collaborate and really communicate well, has been very important in my current role.

Without that clinic experience and the board experience, I honestly don't feel like I would have fostered the amount of leadership skills needed for the roles I play in my current position. In addition, I gained a ton of confidence as well. Thanks to gaining experience right from the start at the clinic where I had to jump right in providing care for someone else.

Wayne Burkholtz (Class of 2010):

Being at the clinic allowed me to get more practice than others who were not a part of the clinic, which was great. The experience was also great because I got a chance to help people and see them get better. PT school is hard, but I was much more interested, much more passionate, because I was able to not just learn but have the opportunity to do.

Christina Wood (Class of 2014):

Being a part of the clinic was a huge part of what guided me to find my job. I also developed my network by attending conferences. At the clinic I was the Clinical Coordinator, so I was in charge of running meetings and making sure that it was running properly, and that all the other members of the pro bono clinic knew what their task was. All these tasks helped me to learn management skills.

Aaron Peffer (Class of 2011):

I think for me it was really an empowering experience just seeing the process of starting a clinic from the ground up with a board of directors essentially that were all students, but all got to have some say in exactly how their little piece played into the whole picture of the clinic. The learning experience has definitely seeped its way into other things I've done, whether it's building programs here at the University of Kentucky, helping their pro bono clinic here, their student-led clinic, and pursuing another degree. It's really set a framework for how I approach those things in terms of working with a team, too. I really took away a lot of great information from the entire experience.

Brian Kennedy (Class of 2015):

I don't think I would understand the intricacies of running a small clinic and what it really takes to motivate the staff which was, you know, our volunteer students and to make sure all those pieces were in place. Where I work is a multidisciplinary setting, with a lot of different professions, a lot of different people working with patients. Having this clinic background, delegating tasks, making sure everyone is on the same page with patients, gave me such a leg up once I got out there.

Jordan Bernstein (Class of 2017):

Without the clinic I probably would not have been as involved as a student at Widener University and also not involved in Chester either. The clinic allowed me to get involved more with the community. I knew very little about Chester prior to the clinic. Without the clinic I also felt that the physical therapy program would not have stood out as much. Being able to provide the experiences and opportunities made it truly special.

Kate Conahan (Class of 2013):

Growing up in a Catholic school all my life, I was a bit sheltered to other religions, cultures, morals, views and being at Widener exposed me to all of that making me a more well-rounded person and connecting with people of all different backgrounds.

Nicole Nardone (Class of 2015):

From the first day you are talking, touching, and treating patients. You are also being mentored by not only second- and third-year students, but also therapists that volunteer their time to work in the clinic. You also get an opportunity to help the community with the services that they really need and gives you a sense of contribution by giving back to those in need.

Widener has always been all about civic engagement, community service, how can you use what you have and what your gifted with to make something sustainable, and that will benefit something else. That clinic really exemplifies it, and the support that both the faculty and just the university in general puts behind the clinic allows us to keep reaching to higher levels. It was a phenomenal once in a lifetime opportunity.

Nicole Rayson (Class of 2016):

The biggest thing that stands out in my mind is the level of competence I have now as a treating clinician starting out. I've only been treating for about half a year now, and there are definitely things that I see in the clinic where I think, "Oh, I've definitely worked with this type of scenario before because I've seen it in the pro bono clinic."

Also, I'd say being in a leadership role really helped me because I am in a position now where I float around to different facilities within this community. Being part of a student board and being part of a large team that took care of a small handful of people at the pro bono clinic has really helped me to manage different team members and having effective communication.

Rich Greenfield (Class of 2012):

I was able to get experience that helped me when it came time to doing my clinical work. PT school is heavily focused on doing group projects, but the clinical work requires you to focus on you and making sure you are ready to be a PT. Going through the clinic I felt I got the experience I needed to feel competent in my work. I cannot place a price or value number on how important those experiences were for me.

Rachel McDermott (Class of 2019):

As a physical therapy student, you can read as much as you want and know your textbooks inside and out, but when it comes to interacting with a patient, it's a completely different ball game. The only thing that prepares you for that is actually doing it, which is why our education through the clinic was so huge. We actually were able to have full-time clinical experiences.

Having the pro bono clinic to start our experience off with the very first summer that we start school is like nothing can compare to that, not only talking to the patients but going through the whole process of having to write a note and having to come up with a plan of care. It's like we knew so much coming into school already, just because we have that experience. You can't get it anywhere else really.

Scott Cheney (Class of 2013):

The leadership that we learned was second to none. Knowing about leadership and doing leadership are two different levels of understanding. Being able to work with others and trust those under you or serving with you was huge. There was also a huge culture built on support. Students were supporting each other, but also the graduating class before would also support. The support did not just stop there, there was help from the community, the school, as well as the professors. This instilled in me a heart for wanting to help others as well.

Another great thing I got at the clinic was being able to start working with patients very early on. Many other programs would not give you a lot of exposure until maybe halfway through your second year. From day one here, you can start treating patients in what you've been trained to do. Now, we are not saying you don't have any supervisor or doing huge major tasks, but you are able to get first-hand experience that jump-starts your learning.

Tim Golder (Class of 2018):

Thanks to the clinic I was able to work on my public speaking skills, presenting on behalf of the clinic at conferences. I also was able to work on my time management skills, which is something many college students struggle with. Lastly, coming into the program I was not really interested in reaching out to the community and volunteering. But my eyes opened up about what was happening in the community especially in Chester, where we were. We got a chance to go ahead and work on providing the needs of those who were in a low socioeconomic area which was a great experience to be a part of.

Final Thoughts

As you can see, the students walked away with far more than your ordinary education in physical therapy. Their skills were greatly enhanced by their time in the clinic. More importantly, they grew as young men and women through service to the community. This personal growth gives the work they do meaning, something money simply cannot buy.

CONCLUSION

As we land the plane on this amazing journey known as "The Widener Experience," I hope you are inspired to think of what is possible for you. This book, as much as it was about a pro bono clinic that was run by students, it was also about leadership, positive working culture, resilience, and community.

For me personally, I study the best companies and organizations such as Apple, Google, Facebook, Airbnb, Lyft, Uber, and Whole Foods, just to name a few, and after learning the pro bono clinic story, I know that Widener is as innovative as these headline companies.

Here are a few of the major takeaways that I believe will serve you as you move forward and build your own careers and programs.

See Them as Their Future

Believe people for what they can be, and not for who they are right now. When I revisit the idea of how faculty didn't want to be referred to as Doctor-this or Mister/Miss-that I realized what the faculty was doing was removing the velvet rope, and letting the students know that they are valued peers. For a student, this validation—which we all seek, whether or not we realize it--is powerful. My jaw still drops thinking about this simple yet effective concept. Friends and colleagues address each other by first names; Widener faculty and students do the same.

If you are reading this right now, I would encourage you to think of ways you can also remove the velvet rope. How do you make people you're engaged with feel like VIPs? If I were a student and my faculty advisors told me to call them by their first name because they already see me as their colleague, I would smile—

right after shedding a tear or reliving the scene from *Pursuit of Happiness* where Will Smith is walking-down the street clapping.

You're More Than Your Title

Another takeaway was the idea of not being limited by your title. Many of the students I interviewed were always open to doing more than what their title entailed. In order for an organization to soar, it needs to know that it is not weighed down by ego-driven people but driven by people who focus on the needs of those they are serving.

The students in this program did not think, "That's XYZ's job, so let them figure it out." Instead, what they did was let the need lead them into moving forward and making things happen. This does not mean everything was perfect, but it does mean that obstacles were seen as problems to be solved. I always like to say you cannot edit a blank page, but if you have something on the page, now you have something to work with.

"The Widener Experience" was exactly that. They did not let what they did not have limit them from thinking what they could have. They were a team in every sense of the word.

There's Power in Purpose

Another takeaway is giving your team something worth believing. When it comes to moving people to act, they must be inspired. The faculty at Widener focused on the needs of the community, and how they could positively impact so many people. As stated in the introduction, so many are unable to receive the proper care needed to have their health restored. This single idea painted a picture that moved students to act. The students were moved, committed, and excited to be a part of helping the people of the Chester community.

The stories of patients who were not able to walk and now could because students actually cared is mind-blowing. The students not only cared, but continued to innovate, improve, and implement year after year. This is the reason why the conferences continue, services are being added, and why many top universities are beginning to implement similar strategies with their various programs to increase impact and effectiveness.

The Greatest Teacher is Experience

One last takeaway that merits mentioning is what the students were able to become as a result of the opportunities this student-run model afforded them. Many students were able to improve decision making skills, maximize resources, and build confidence as they moved into their careers. This is essentially what graduate school is supposed to be: a sneak preview of what real life is like.

With the clinic, the students did not have to wait for those opportunities because they were already facing them head on. This is something that makes the physical therapy program at Widener and similar universities invaluable to prospective students.

Being a first-year PT student with real-world work experience was a confidence booster for the Widener students when interacting with other students and professionals at conferences, as well as during clinical education experiences. These are the kind of opportunities this model produced.

This conclusion could be the topic of a second book, so it is best we stop here.

Realize this important fact: Inspiration is great, but not greater than implementation. Intentions are good but are worthless if not acted upon. The information in this book serves no one if nothing changes.

There are clients whose health and function were at stake and students waiting to be challenged, waiting to rise to the occasion and show what they are made of. Miracles do not happen if our comfort zones are not disturbed, so faculty reading this should be confident and comfortable even when facing rough waters. As stated by Franklin D Roosevelt: "A smooth sea never made a skillful sailor."

Go ahead and challenge yourself to figure out how you can empower, encourage, and enlarge the capacities of the students you are called to lead. This is the mark of a great teacher—providing experiences that enable students to learn about the profession first hand, and not just read about it.

One final thought: Please do not keep this book to yourself. Share it with your colleagues. Also, please do not limit it to just physical therapy. While we did talk about how Widener went from having no clinic to the clinic that is hosting conferences on both coasts of the United States, this book is so much more than that. It's really about the power of students when they are given the opportunity to fail. It's only because of that opportunity that they can also experience the joy of success. This lesson is something all students can benefit from, regardless of their field of study.

Our dream is to create a culture where students are more hands-on and trusted with more. Transitioning to this culture will feel weird at first. There will be awkward moments and there will be bumping of heads, but the end result—the skilled, confident graduates—will make it all worthwhile.

Thank you for your attention on this journey with us. I look forward to reading about the experiences you will create.

THE IMAGES BEHIND
"THE WIDENER EXPERIENCE"

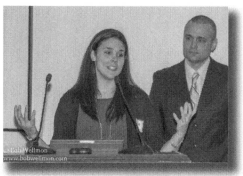

Christina Guay

(Class of 2014 Clinic Coordinator)
It was her idea to start the conferences, the first of which was
held in March 2013. Scott Cheney (2013 Clinic Coordinator.)
to her left was the first Widener student to serve on the Board of
the Society for Student-Run Free Clinics.

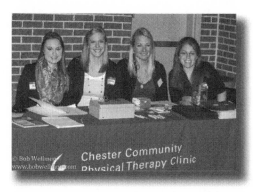

From L-R: Alie Ferguson, Elizabeth Long, Stephanie Mielach,
Elya Spolar. Pro Bono Network Conference 2013.

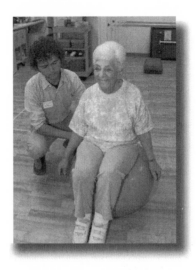

Aaron Peffer (Class of 2011; Community Relations/Marketing Officer) working with the clinic's second client. She had fractured her ankle from a fall and had exhausted her Medicare benefit for the year. Aaron is challenging her balance to help prevent future falls.

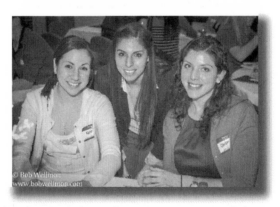

Katie D'Ambrosia (Class of 2015 Community Relations and Marketing Officer); Alanna DiBiaisi (Class of 2015 Fund Officer); Christine Solomon (Class of 2014 Community Relations and Marketing Officer).

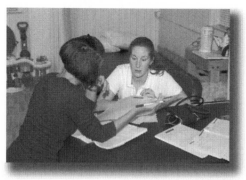

Melissa Higgins (R) and Lauren Davidson (L) conferring and documenting after client care ended. Both are Student Board members from the Class of 2011.

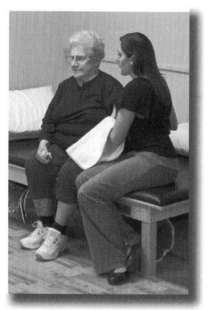

Vanessa Kershaw (Class of 2011 Fund Officer) working with a client. Kershaw launched the first 5K fundraiser.

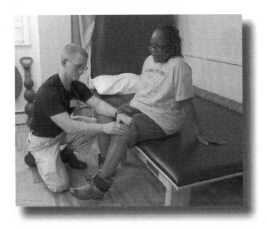

Chris Carroll (Class of 2014 Fund Officer) with Rev. Regina
Goodrich (community leader and now serves on the clinic's
Community Advisory Board). Chris took the 5K and grew it to
a whole new level.

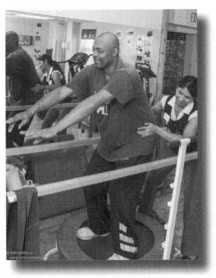

Meghan Jacob (Class of 2015 Client Advocate) working with a
client in the parallel bars.

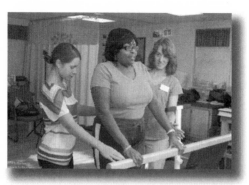

Jen Ogden (Class of 2015 Health and Wellness Coordinator) and Caitlin Grobaker (Class of 2016 Fund Officer) working on balance activities with a client.

Pro Bono Network Conference – group of students from Thomas Jefferson University who presented.

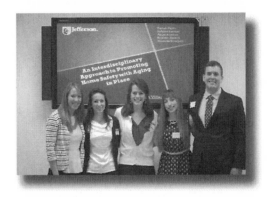

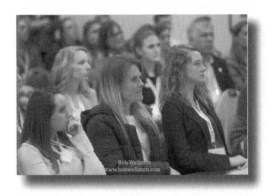

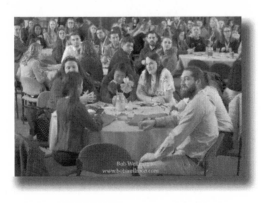

"The Widener Experience"

Eastern Regional Conference 2018

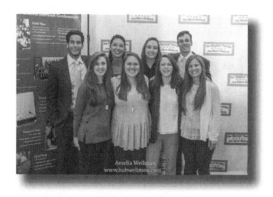

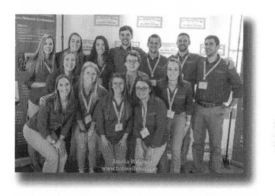

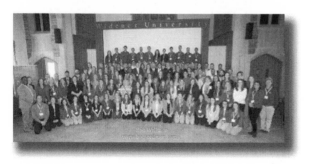

Western Conference 2018 – Northern Arizona University

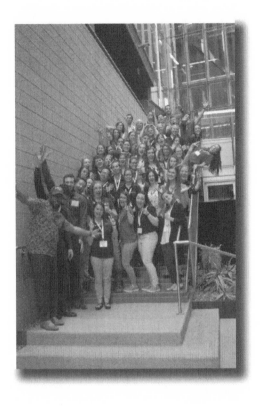

STUDENT LEADERSHIP

Class of 2021

Clinic Coordinator: John Nellet
National Honor Society Officer: Haily Vaka
National Conference Chair: Alyssa Myers
Marketing Officer: John Vizzini and Rachel Pisarra
Student Relations: Brittany Erlsten
Fund Officers: Emily Swope and Rachael DiGuglielmo
Outcomes Coordinator: Megan McCurdy
Operations Coordinator: Josh Hammaker
Alumni Relations: Stephanie Saylor
Health and Wellness Coordinator: Danielle Hemerka
Client Advocate: Gabrielle Crespo
Social Media Marketing Officer: Eva Reyes

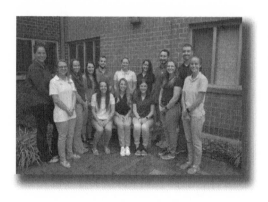

Class of 2020

Clinic Coordinator: David Aurand
National Honor Society Officer: Baylee Mann
National Conference Chair: Alaina Curry
Marketing Officer: Troy Koch and Zach Shustyk
Student Relations: Kimmy Hall
Fund Officers: Kayla Herr and Katie Sterling
Outcomes Coordinator: Taylor Stone
Operations Coordinator: Max Schrom
Alumni Relations: Andrea Barajas
Health and Wellness Coordinator: Beth Pirtle
Client Advocate: Laura Giordano
Social Media Marketing Officer: Joe Ruszkowski

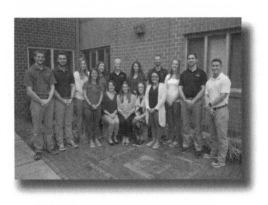

Class of 2019

Clinic Coordinator: Justin Gilfillan
National Honor Society Officer: Rachel McDermott
National Conference Chair: Jonathan Rouse
Marketing Officer: Patrick Rutledge
Student Relations: Amanda Schmidt
Fund Officers: Elizabeth Antonucci, Leo Harmon, and Jacqueline Ruggiero
Outcomes Coordinator: Taylor Stone
Operations Coordinator: Reed Hoffman
Alumni Relations: Jaclyn Krempasky
Health and Wellness Coordinator: Kristine Sindoni
Client Advocate: Kathleen Flynn
Social Media Marketing Officer: Heather Burns

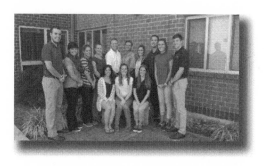

Class of 2018

Clinic Coordinator: Tim Golder
National Honor Society Officer: Brianna Englert
National Conference Chair: Jenna Newton
Marketing Officers: Mike Berardo and Jordan Bernstein
Student Relations: Danielle Bazalek
Fund Officers: Brittany Burkholder and Kasey Dietrich
Outcomes Coordinator: Tyler Suruskie
Operations Coordinator: Seth Brakefield
Alumni Relations: Liz Langer
Health and Wellness Coordinator: Steve Grazioli
Client Advocate: Nicolina Marcela
Social Media Marketing Officer: Kristina Reiter

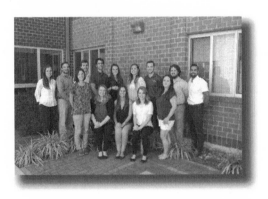

Class of 2017

Clinic Coordinator: Nolan Converse
National Honor Society Officer: Maggie Karmens
National Conference Chair: Melinda Berean
Student Relations: Kristen Luer
Fund Officers: Kristen French
Outcomes Coordinator: Kyle Hughes
Operations Coordinator: Zach Mease
Alumni Relations: Lauren Oxford
Health and Wellness Coordinator: Mike Fernandez
Client Advocate: Khyati Shah
Social Media Marketing Officer: Kaitlyn Schnaulzer

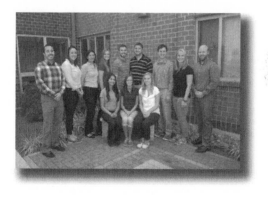

Class of 2016

Clinic Coordinator: Daria Poretta
Community Relations Officer: Sleby Weiss
Marketing Officer: Nicole Rayson
Fund Officer: Caitlin Grobaker
Outcomes Coordinator: Kerry McIntyre
Operations Coordinator: Jon Bellizio
Alumni Relations: Sarah Voelkel
Health and Wellness Coordinator: Kyle Bauer and Georgia Spano
Client Advocate: Amy Albano

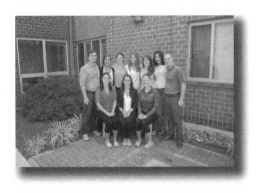

Class of 2015

Clinic Coordinator: Brian Kennedy
Community Relations Officer: Katherine D'Ambrosia
Marketing Officer: Dale Jones
Fund Officers: Alanna DiBiasi, Elizabeth Long
Student Relations: Haelim Park
Outcomes Coordinator: Nicole Nardone, Jessica Pierce
Operations Coordinator: Jonathan Dwyer
Alumni Relations: Meghan Jacob
Health and Wellness Coordinator: Rebekah Coleman, Jennifer Ogden
Client Advocate: Nicole Gezzi

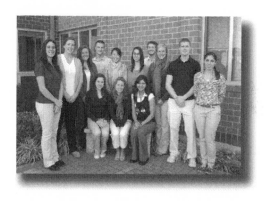

Class of 2014

Clinic Coordinator: Christina Guay
Community Relations Officer: Courtney Christman
Marketing Officer: Christine Solomon
Fund Officer: Chris Carroll
Student Relations: Alexandra Ferguson
Outcomes Coordinator: Stephanie Zerhusen
Operations Coordinator: Jacob Daniels
Alumni Relations: Josh Houseal
Health and Wellness Coordinator: Joe Connor
Client Advocate: Stephanie Mielach

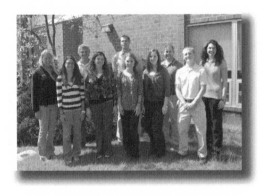

Class of 2013

Clinic Coordinator: Scott Cheney
Community Relations Officer: John Ohlaver
Marketing Officer: Theresa Lennon
Fund Officer: Jeff Cain
Student Relations: Holly Green
Outcomes Coordinator: Kate Conahan
Operations Coordinator: Amanda Ott, Lauren Papps
Alumni Relations: Dana Calderoni
Client Advocate: Karen Hemmes

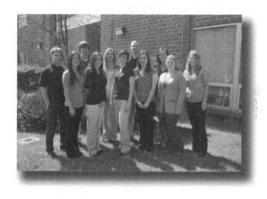

Class of 2012

Clinic Coordinator: Caitlin Kirkpatrick
Community Relations Officer: Jon Herting
Fund Officer: Michael Root
Student Relations: Jaime Cafaro
Outcomes Coordinator: Erica Melfe
Operations Coordinator: Nate Haas
Alumni Relations: Richard Greenfield
Client Relations: Jordan Shettle

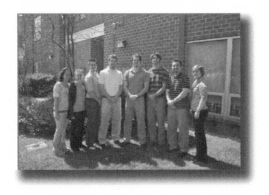

Class of 2011

Clinic Coordinator: Melinda Agarwal
Community Relations Officer: Aaron Peffer
Fund Officer: Vanessa Kershaw
Student Relations: Lauren Davidson
Outcomes Coordinator: Jess Darrah and Melissa Higgins
Operations Coordinator: Amanda Reinmiller and Allecia Langston
Alumni Relations: Christina Flasinski
Client Relations: Mallory Meyer

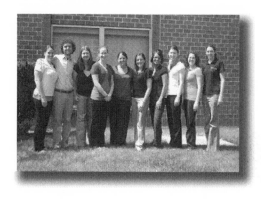

Class of 2010

Clinic Coordinator: Beth Sander
Community Relations Officer: Wayne Burkholtz and Charlie Moore
Fund Officer: Heather Wnorowski and Kim Herbertson
Student Relations: Danielle Rosen
Outcomes Coordinator: Amber Bennick
Operations Coordinator: Crystal Ayers and Tony Sacerino
Alumni Relations: Heather Goldy
Client Relations: Jen Hardy

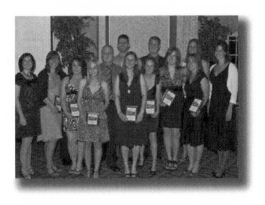